Behavioral Types
and
The Art Of Patient Management

Improving Quality of Care With
Better Understanding Of
Physician-Patient Relationships

Stephen E. Prather, M.D.
Robert R. Blake, Ph.D.
Jane S. Mouton, Ph.D.

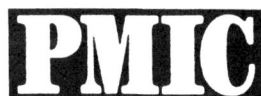

Library of Congress Cataloging-in-Publication Data

Prather, Stephen E.
    Behavioral types and the art of patient management : improving quality of care with better understanding of physician-patient relationships / Stephen E. Prather, Robert R. Blake, and Jane S. Mouton.
        p. cm.
Originally published as: Medical risk management, 1990.
Includes bibliographical references and index.
        ISBN 1-57066-031-X
1.Physician and patient. 2. Repertory grid technique.
I. Blake, Robert Rogers, 1918- . II. Mouton, Jane Srygley.
III. Prather, Stephen E. Medical risk management. IV. Title.
R727.P73 1995   95-16790
610.69'6--dc20   CIP

ISBN 1-57066-031-X

The Grid® is a registered trademark of Scientific Methods, Inc., P.O. Box 195, Austin, TX 78767.

Practice Management Information Corp. (PMIC)
4727 Wilshire Blvd., Suite 300
Los Angeles, CA 90010

Printed in the United States of America

DISCLAIMER
This publication is designed to provide accurate and authoritative information in regard to the subject matter covered. It is sold with the understanding that the publisher is not engaged in rendering legal, accounting, or other professional service. If professional, personal or other expert assistance is required, the services of a competent professional should be sought. Though all of the information contained herein has been carefully researched and checked for accuracy and completeness, neither the authors nor the publisher accept any responsibility or liability with regard to errors, omissions, misuse, or misinterpretation.

DEDICATION

Dr. Jane Mouton died unexpectedly on December 7, 1987, as an earlier version of this manuscript was being written. Since it represents her initiative in originating Grid development and the culmination of her 35-year devotion to enriching it, this book is dedicated in her memory.

ACKNOWLEDGMENT

Appreciation is extended to Helen Hodgson, Ph.D., president of Health/Life Planning, Inc., who provided a vast amount of insight and contribution to this work as editor and consultant throughout the development of the "Caring for Difficult Patients" program.

This text is the basis for the "Mastering Medical Care: Redefining Physician Leadership" seminar, which focuses on the concept of physician excellence described in this book. The seminar is copyrighted by Scientific Methods, Inc., and is conducted exclusively by Medical Resource Management, 505 East 200 South, Suite 302, Salt Lake City, Utah 84102.

CONTENTS

PREFACE

Patients — some say a majority of them — are becoming increasingly difficult to care for. As medicine has grown in complexity, so have the patients. The physician has become more discontent and more threatened than ever before, even though patients have never lived longer or with less suffering. The answer to this crisis in job satisfaction is obviously tied to lost autonomy, declining reimbursement, malpractice allegations, and a declining public image. More fundamentally than that, though, it lies in the fact that medicine today is critically different from that of the past. The difference is one of expectations. Society, patients, and physicians are caught up in miscommunication and conflicts brought on by the unrealistic expectations of everyone involved. Physicians face a loss of patient trust and a loss of control, an unexpected situation that is unprecedented in modern medicine.

The problem is in the traditional physician-patient model, which is based on the relationship of an expert working with a novice. In the past, this relationship often created a childlike dependency in adult patients. However, even when resentment resulted, it did not obstruct the delivery of care because the relationship was based on trust and the physician was the final authority. Now, if the expectation of a perfect outcome is not met, it is viewed by the patient as a case of poor-quality care; and this, coupled with dependency, leads to resentment, which can manifest itself in medical malpractice lawsuits. This situation demands physicians learn new skills of professional interdependence and avoid the potential negative dynamics of the old model of physician-patient interaction.

In record numbers, physicians have been searching for a new approach as a solution to these crisis times. Many are forming groups in order to build strategies. One option has been to concede to the new "corporatization" of medicine and trade in the professional ethic for a business contract and cookbook solutions based on categorized diagnoses and standardized treatments. Another "quick fix" solution has been to improve appearances by redecorating the office, starting a newsletter, and, of course, advertising. Neither approach has any impact on improving the quality of care. The challenge of mastering medical care, as you will see, is significant. Part of the challenge involves redefining clinical leadership.

This book is dedicated to those physicians and health professionals who are willing to meet the challenges presented by the new business of health care delivery. But more than that, it is for those who also remain committed to creating the highest quality of care by raising the level of trust and communication with patients and peers, even those who are the most difficult. The highest quality medical care that can be achieved is only possible through a structure that allows those who are committed to undertake a lifetime of continuous improvement, no matter what the challenge. The focus of this book is on your ability to create the patient of the future, who must learn to make cost-efficient decisions while assuming shared responsibility with you, the care provider. This patient must also understand the limits of medical practice, in terms of procedures as well as expected results; perfect outcomes cannot be guaranteed, even with the highest quality care. By acquiring a particular style of physician leadership, you can create the atmosphere required to face the challenge of the new and more difficult circumstances you will face in the future. It will always fall to the physician to instill realistic patient expectations, to encourage self-responsibility, and to ensure the highest technical quality possible, Only then can we begin the recovery process of a health care system presently on the verge of financial disaster.

A scientifically based body of work directed toward these goals has never before existed in the field of medicine. The Grid concept presented here, adapted to medicine in 1985, has been used for more than 30 years in investigating sound and unsound practices in basic human relationships. Applied to clinical circumstances, it has been shown to decrease claims frequency of physicians who have received multiple lawsuits and significantly impacts the performance of complex clinical teams. The Grid is also cross cultural. Used in industry, government, sales, universities, and even domestic situations, the Grid has proven its widespread applicability in many parts of the world. This tool, applied to the intensive and emergency care areas of the hospital, has helped physicians direct a team through a crisis in much the same way that this concept has been successfully adapted for use in cockpit flight simulations and used by pilots to deal with life-threatening crises in the air. The leadership skills stressed in the Grid are essential for effectively mobilizing human resources to ensure that the highest quality results can be obtained in any highly charged, high-risk career. The experience gained with over 7,000 pilots, whose incentive for excellence is literally their own lives as well as the lives of the millions who take to the airways, demonstrated dramatic improvements in key performance parameters. Risk management research, which provides the underpinning of this work, has shown that these same leadership skills are equally important to physicians in primary care, surgical amphitheaters, intensive care units, emergency rooms, and labor and delivery suites.

High-risk situations in a high-stakes medical-legal environment require problem solving, decision making, supportive teamwork, and clear communication under pressure. This is what mastering medical care is all about. Documented decreases in claims frequency and dollars lost in litigation have been the measurable reward for those physicians who have taken this approach. Additional benefits have been peace of mind and a new ability to participate as a clinical leader. This new skill has become a requirement for success in the new and complex systems of health care delivery.

The Grid framework depicted in this book provides a greater understanding of the most common leadership styles used in medicine and clarifies which ones can ensure excellence, even when challenged by the truly difficult patient in the most difficult situations. It is a mirror to help physicians and other care providers in analyzing themselves and a guide to building new practice skills. Each medical management style is detailed to clarify its pitfalls and to provide the motivation for changing practice styles. Even though this material is helpful to the entire medical team, it focuses on practical applications for the physician who is "running the practice" and leading the team.

This book has been designed for physicians in all specialties of medicine, as well as for those other members of the medical team who will benefit from its approach. The first chapter offers an overview and points out that meeting the needs of difficult patients requires a concern that must be equally balanced between the human needs of each patient and the technical expertise required to obtain the highest quality outcome from medical care. In the second chapter, the physician begins to identify a personal Grid style. This new insight regarding style is carried into Chapter 3, which reveals the impact of the patient's Grid style on the physician-patient interaction.

Chapters 4 to 9 detail the six major physician styles, pointing out the pitfalls and benefits of each and indicating how various patients respond to each of these physicians. Six elements of leadership, all of which are interdependent, define a progression of medical care: 1) *Communication* is essential to 2) *acquiring knowledge,* both of which underlie 3) *decision making.* After a decision is made, 4) *initiative* determines how the medical care will be delivered. Conflicts, either within the medical team or between the physician and patient, may then arise. At this point, 5) *conflict resolution* becomes critical. The final step, which may be the most important for quality assurance as well as risk prevention, is ongoing 6) *critique and feedback.* Motivations to change and rewards for successfully moving into the style of practice that is most likely to meet the needs of all of the professionals involved in care and all types of patients are clear by the end of Chapter 9.

Chapter 10 details the phases of what could become a medical revolution. This revolution would be built on a new concept in physician-led teamwork integrated into a system of care that could result in the same financial and personal rewards already demonstrated by the use of these new skills in other high-risk professions.

Appendix A expands the ideas of the text with an overview of the central challenge that faces us all. It considers the issues of truly mastering our own personal approach to one-on-one relationships, interdependent professional groups, delivering care, and the new integrated health care delivery systems.

In a profession currently under attack, you, the individual physician, find yourself entangled in complex changes that are largely beyond your control.

However, regardless of the turmoil created by shifts in societal expectations, government regulations, and, most importantly, the business of health care delivery, medicine remains a critically important profession, and you, the physician, possess the key to achieving the highest quality care by mastering the skills described here.

This book is not the sole answer to America's health care crisis, but it is a major personal step toward positive growth and a rebuilding of the professional ideals for which you stand.

Chapter One

THE GRID APPROACH
TO MEDICAL EXCELLENCE

The gray, wet cold filled the parking lot as Dr. Thomas Jones pulled up to the gate where his magnetic passcard allowed entry to a narrow channel winding its way between filled parking spaces. As he found the only remaining space, in front of the door clearly marked fire zone, *he thought, "How can the hospital keep adding staff without being able to provide parking, let alone patients, for them?"*

Even though he had just eaten, his stomach groaned for food. His mind was on another cup of coffee, which might have justified the agitation and impatience he felt sweep over him.

It was 30 minutes before his first patient in the office, and with five patients to round on, he would be just a little late. But that would be okay; he would call the office so the patients would know he was caught in the hospital. Maybe then he could find a parking space — if they hadn't already towed his car away.

Mrs. Tanner, the patient in 278, had asked him to plan on extra time this morning. He wondered if she was upset with the postop infection or the long stay. "Have I spent enough time with her? That's always such a difficult question to answer, but she'll be fine. She's going home today."

He moved for the handle on the door, feeling his stomach relax, remembering as the day actually got underway that he would get into the flow of his practice and see the answers and make the right decisions. Then he thought, "It'll be a long day, a full office, another PPO members' meeting to discuss some physician who continually refuses to use the hospital ultrasound department under the new health plan. And, of course, there is always call — being available, losing sleep. The cramps in the abdomen will return tonight, on call, when most are asleep."

He moved into the hospital only to hear, "Dr. Jones, Dr. Thomas Jones." Already a modification of how the day had been mentally rehearsed. He picked up the phone.

"Doctor, oh my God, get to labor and delivery! Your patient is bleeding, and we can't get heart tones."

"What patient?"

1

"She just came in. I don't remember her name. I've got an IV in, and anesthesia is here. We are in real trouble!"

"Move her to the C-section room. Get some blood; I'm on my way.

The pace picked up. A fullness filled his chest as color returned to cheeks chilled by the oppressive winter smog; a looseness began to enter his shoulders. He was instantly ready to take in all the facts and respond to the circumstances he faced. There was no hunger, no fear-only control, as he pulled all of the steps together to make a sound decision under fire. The fathers' waiting room was in a panic; obviously the seriousness of the situation had reached the family. They all knew exactly who he was by the speed in his step.

"Oh, Dr. Jones, she's dying!"

*He slowed to a stop; he reached out his hand and forced a handshake with the woman he imagined to be the grandmother. "Of course, the situation is serious, but we're doing our best. I want you to sit down and keep everybody calm. You've been through childbirth and so you know what it's like. It **always** seems scary; but we have seen this situation before, and we are doing everything possible to help her. I will be back as soon as I can."*

Dr. Jones had taken 10 seconds of the time that separated him from the dressing room and beginning surgery on a woman quite likely to be in shock. He had not spoken with any quiver in his voice and had talked appropriately fast. It was clear that he was concerned but confident.

Gowned in surgical scrubs, he saw a trail of blood leading to the operating room where the father was standing outside the door. As he passed the nurses' station, Dr. Jones glanced at the chart to identify the patient. She was at term, was mildly anemic, and had a risk score of zero. That was all he had time to see, except for the patient's and husband's names. This was only the second time he had met the husband, who was in tears, but was not crying, not moving, and not able to understand.

"Jim, I've got to hurry. Time is important, but as soon as we are done, I will come out and tell you what is going on. I'm sorry you can't come in. Julie will be asleep, and we are doing all we can. Here, sit down, Jim. We are going to do our best to see that your wife is okay. The nurses have already gotten everything started."

Dr. Jones turned and signaled the ward clerk to help him. Jim was crying now, and he needed to sit down. Dr. Jones blasted through the door to see the patient and assess the situation.

Vital signs were unstable. He glanced at the blood type and reviewed the fetal monitor tracing. Julie's legs were strapped firmly in place. She was still conscious and oddly stoic and strong. "What's wrong, Dr. Jones?"

He offered reassurance. "We're going to be moving pretty fast here, Julie; but with all this bleeding, you're going to need a C-section. Jim is outside, and he knows what is going on. You're going to go to sleep now." He waited for a nod of recognition.

"Is my baby all right?"

"I hope so, Julie. We will do our best. Try to relax." He looked up. *"How much time?"*

The anesthesiologist said, *"Whenever you're ready, Dr. Jones."*

"We had better get going, Julie. I'm just going to wash my hands." As he turned out of earshot from the patient, he asked, *"How much blood loss?"* The nurse replied, *"2000 cc."*

He frowned as he paused to reevaluate the situation, *"She wouldn't still be awake if she'd lost 2000 cc's. Did anybody check her?"*

"No."

"Is she in labor?"

"I don't think so."

"Can you get heart tones?" The nurse did not reply, but simply shook her head no.

He moved back to Julie to see if she was still alert. *"We are going to wash your stomach now."* Tom spoke softly as he gestured for the circulator to begin the prep. *"Don't worry, Julie, we do this all the time."* He caught her eye, and under the mask, she could see him smiling.

As he turned back to the circulator, his voice was more firm. *"I want this baby out in 4 minutes; it is 8:37. We don't have time to listen to the fetal heart tones. Prep the abdomen, and put her down. Is there anything else I need to know?"*

"No, you have all of the information we have. Should I get a pediatrician?" she asked.

"You get started here. I'll take care of it."

Tom moved to the scrub room where he met the resident assistant, just finishing up her scrub. *"We've really got to move on this one. Get in there and get her draped. I want this baby out in 3 minutes. She's got a Foley in place. We're ready to go. She'll probably be in shock by the time we get in. Don't say anything until she is asleep, and don't touch her abdomen after she's draped. She's scared, and I don't want her thinking that we have started the case before she's asleep. Any questions?"* She shook her head no and moved through the doors to the operating room.

He began a 30-second scrub with the bristle side of the brush. He took a breath and reviewed the case in his mind. What might not be there? Instruments, the bulb syringe; oh yes, a pediatrician.

He looked up and hit the intercom. *"Barbara, call pediatrics and get someone here now.*

She replied, *"Do you know who the pediatrician is?"*

"It's on the admit sheet, but I need someone now. This baby is in trouble."

He moved to the operating room, checked the Mayo stand. All the instruments were there. He looked at the blood as he finished draping the patient. The anesthesiologist looked up. *"Okay, you can cut."*

Two minutes later, a lifeless, pale infant was born. The pediatric nurses began resuscitation. Barbara came over the intercom. "Dr. Wheeler will be in. He is changing."

"Set up for a UAC" was the verbal order from the obstetrician whose experience told him the baby would require a central line.

"We usually let the pediatrician make that decision, Dr. Jones. I think we had better take the baby to the nursery.

"Set up for a UAC now. Call the nursery and tell Dr. Wheeler we need him now." He passed a second ring clamp to the assistant and asked for suture to be loaded.

"Do we have Pitocin running? I want 2 grams of antibiotic, STAT. Stitch."

The pediatrician came through the door. Dr. Jones didn't look up. "Kenny, there was no blood in the cord; you've got an abruption."

The pediatrician quickly intubated the infant, who was beginning to respond. "I need a UAC."

"It's right here, doctor."

The bleeding was under control, and Dr. Jones turned to the anesthesiologist. "Okay, what's our pressure? Get 2 units of blood. It's looking good here, Kenny. How's the baby?"

"Real trouble. We need to transfer this one. Get me the university."

"Any heart rate?" Tom asked.

"Yeah, but that's about it. Give me some more normal saline, and get some blood up here."

The pediatrician looked over his shoulder. "We got the line in, Tom."

The surgery finished well. The Apgars were discouraging at 1, 3, and 5; but by the time of the transfer, the blood was in and spontaneous movement and breathing had returned. And there were no seizures — yet.

As Dr. Jones took off his gown, he said, "We really worked as a team. Everybody did a great job; I'm glad you kept so cool." He then thanked everyone, addressing most by their first names. He shook the circulator's hand and then turned to the scrub nurse. "Now that was fast. I feel we did all we could." Turning to the anesthesiologist, "Great anesthesia. Was there anything we could have done differently to make this kind of thing easier for anyone?"

Jean, the circulator, looked up and said, "Yeah, pass out valium." Everyone laughed and agreed that they had really gotten it together.

Dr. Jones moved to the hall. He approached the husband and family in a warm, caring, sympathetic way. He was relaxed and confident, thanks to the positive feedback and laughter that the surgical team had taken the time to share. No one would believe that only minutes before he had been bathed with blood to his elbows. Tom was realistic with the family but he gave them hope. "The baby will get the very best care in the newborn intensive care unit, and they can do amazing things." Jim couldn't help but cry.

Tom stayed with the family, relaying messages for the transport team until

Julie was awake. When he returned to Julie, he smiled and told her that she was okay and that the baby was doing well, considering everything she had gone through. She smiled and thanked him; and a tear nearly came to his eye, knowing the rough road ahead for all of them.

Dr. Jones turned back to the changing room and dressed, ready to face his office. He wondered if it would be overcrowded with patients who didn't have time to sit around and wait. He reflected on how his office nurse could reschedule his day. "Rounds will be made at lunch, and the afternoon office schedule will also need to be adjusted so that I don't fall behind."

On his way out of the hospital, he stopped by to tell Mrs. Tanner of the emergency and that he hadn't forgotten her.

The cold, damp weather was just as oppressive when he left the hospital, but somehow Tom was no longer able to see it that way. That day he was the best. He was a true physician; and if any human potential was meant for the baby, he had done all that was possible to achieve it. Because communication had been handled well, the family was able to understand what had happened. The mother had lived, and Dr. Jones himself would recover easily from the minor complaints and criticisms he would face in the office.

He stood at the crosswalk, calmly waiting for the red light to change. His stomach felt good. The anticipation of the long day was behind him. His day had begun well.

Defining Clinical Leadership

Was the highest quality result achieved? Did Dr. Jones get sued? The answers to these questions are at least partly based on just how difficult a style Julie had. If you say she was not difficult at all, then you underestimate the tremendous emotional impact that a damaged baby can have on a mother. Less-than-perfect outcomes make a patient difficult to care for, especially now when a lawyer is eager to take her case before a sympathetic jury. If you felt her style made her low risk to care for, then remember that Dr. Jones had 9 months to evaluate and modify her style prior to the episode that you just reviewed. All specialties are not so lucky, yet obstetrics remains at the forefront of medical-legal jeopardy and is the focus of a nationwide quality assurance probe.

The difficult patient may demonstrate one of several leadership styles. With a poor outcome, in this case a bad baby, the patient may become an enigma because a back-up style that is only seen under stress may surface. If a patient wants to make a win-lose battle out of the conflicts that naturally occur as a result of less-than-perfect outcomes, then he or she will become even more difficult to care for and the quality of future care may suffer.

What is Dr. Jones' role? What impact did he have on this patient's style?

What effect did he have on the clinical team? Has he ever encouraged patients to seek care elsewhere because their style made them too high risk to care for? The answers to these questions are keys to developing the medical leadership demanded by this new era in patient care.

Every doctor, regardless of specialty, age, or location, has a dominant practice style that reflects his or her ability to lead, care for patients, and work with all of the personnel necessary for high-quality medical care. In the current medical-legal climate, and with increasing regulation and competition, many physicians have been looking for short-term solutions to this seeming crisis of confidence. Some have now resorted to survival tactics. They have lost sight of the fact that leadership is the most significant factor in success or failure of their practice.

Strong and effective leadership is expressed in many ways and is essential in achieving the best medical results. High-quality medical care stimulates the patient to participate in the healing process, purchase our services, and accept the fact that we cannot always guarantee a perfect outcome.

In addition to the medical skills called on, a foundation in trust is needed by the entire medical management team. To achieve this, it is essential that team members have a shared commitment and a clear sense of purpose. They must give one another mutual support, by understanding and respecting each other's perspectives, even when they differ.

To achieve the highest quality outcomes during the current crisis in medicine, physicians must master new skills of cooperation. They must demand excellence from themselves and from those who help them deliver medical care. If physicians are to meet the needs of society, patients must be stimulated to participate in their care and to begin to share responsibility in the outcome — good or bad.

This book provides principles critical to mastering medical care by clarifying what effective leadership is and by contrasting it with alternative ways of exercising leadership that miss the mark of excellence. It can help you direct your own programs to achieve clinical practice improvement by eliminating barriers to clinical teamwork and ensuring effectiveness when faced with difficult patients. The best way to use this book is to compare the principles that define each of the six Grid styles with your own ways of practicing. As you review Dr. Jones' story, ask yourself how you respond to a medical crisis. "Do I exhibit this kind of leadership in my practice?" As each Grid style is presented, consider, "Do I do this?" "Should I be more (or less) like this type of physician?"

This book permits you to locate your practice style on a Grid. Once you have found your unique place, Grid principles become a guide to encourage you to be more self-analytical during the ongoing challenge provided by the needs of patients. The first goal is to strengthen your communication and leadership skills. Then you can be more effective in an environment in which you sell your services (medical care), work with colleagues, and direct and manage other medical team members (nurses, extenders, therapists, administrators). All are important because each impacts significantly on patients in an arena of disease and health, pain and suffering, and life and death that has no parallel elsewhere in life. You must be an investigator, teacher, counselor, promoter, and, of course, diligent medical practitioner. But above all else, you must be a leader. The second goal, which complements the first, is to learn to recognize the high-risk situation before it occurs. You must understand the styles of the patients who face you as well as those of the members of your team in order to build strategies that will ensure your success no matter what the clinical outcome.

You're Not Alone

The methodology that we have described for providing optimal care for difficult patients rests on an understanding of cultural change. We have made a rapid transit from a broad, culture-centered perspective, seen in preliterate societies, through a culture that reinforced compliance with reward, to what is now once again a broad, culture-centered perspective for an entirely new reason.

A brief review of anthropological research reveals that preliterate times were regulated by customs. Behavior is assumed to have been generally subject to free choice and, at its best, organized in a system consistent with an orientation of involvement and commitment predicated on shared decision making and limited only by the individual skills and intelligence of the societal member. Communication is assumed to have been face to face by word of mouth, and hunters and gatherers likely made their decisions as equals by consensus. A dominant individual became the leader, again by consensus.

What evolved with the development of language-organized societies and a reward system, which differentiated roles, identified certain jobs as "more valuable," and allowed monies to be accumulated so that material possessions could be "owned" in an era of surplus, stimulated what we have described in this book as a 9+9 or paternalistic separation of what had previously been inseparable. With the shift from hunting to herding and from picking to planting somewhere between the 12th and 10th century B.C., laws were laid down and military institutions were developed that had clear-cut figures of authority. The rearing of children, education, the penal system, and much of what became organized religion adopted a paternalistic style of leadership. The societal control exhibited by paternalistic techniques, although resulting in a bloody resolution of differences, provided an understandable framework, which has persisted into the modern era. No doubt one of the fundamental reasons for its success was its deep rooting in the basic religious model of what was and often still is presumed to be a sound relationship between God and man. "Not my will but Thine be done..." is a paternalistic precept by which the speaker relinquishes self-responsibility. Action was based not on what he or she wished or thought to be right, but rather on what religious authority said was correct and proper. In a society where impoverishment and poor sanitation were the norm and where life expectancy was short, the carnage of childbirth extreme, and the visible earthly reward limited, people were sustained by the strong traditional belief that reward for compliance was withheld until the hereafter — a time free of the poverty, hunger, and deprivation that characterized the long, bitter battle of life. Was this paternalistic model accepted because of its soundness or because people needed greater rewards and deeper sources of security than life was able to offer?

Regardless of the answer to that question, it is clear that today, in the "modern era," a great change is underway. Perhaps escalated by the materialism and affluence that came in the aftermath of World War II, people have simply become less dependent on a leader's discretion in providing external rewards, particularly now that the reward is so often measured in dollars and cents. People are less fearful of suffering financial deprivation than they once were of suffering damnation for noncompliance with leadership direction.

One of the most dramatic examples of a rebellion against paternalistic leadership in the United States occurred in education during the 1960s, with the successful resistance of college students to the *in loco parentis* orientation of academic administrations. Students throughout the school system became far less willing to do what the teacher required in exchange for grades and promotion to the next level. At the same time, the institution of marriage, although vowed before God, family, and friends, and based on rules laid down centuries before, was taking on the character of a contractual relationship. Husbands and wives refused to maintain marriages that had meaning only in terms of the promised reward for compliance, if the relationships were no longer based on understanding and fulfillment.

Accepting these shifts in values as real, and suspending our judgment about the good or bad direction they have taken, leads to an important conclusion: Society cannot and will not reestablish voluntary order by moving in the direction of increased paternalism. Yet it is this system that created medicine.

Its limitation in the eyes of society is vividly demonstrated by once-appreciative patients suing their physicians in record numbers. This breakdown in the traditional relationship of caring and trust is the primary reason that society has felt the need to begin its own evaluation of the quality of medical care we deliver. Profiles on quality outcomes are already in place, allowing a comparison of physician against physician and hospital against hospital. This is the real incentive to implement your own program to meet the patient's needs and the public's expectations in an era when societal change has made your job so much more difficult. The skills needed to master medical care in this new era are simple enough in intellectual terms, but mastering the behavior requisite to open cooperative leadership, communication, conflict resolution, and critique is another matter. This leadership orientation emphasizes sound teamwork as a process of interaction based on openness and candor, thorough inquiry, effective decision making, strong initiative, creative conflict solving, and two-way critique. To master these skills in medical care, you must answer an important question: "How do I make this a part of my life?"

Your first step will be to determine whether or not you feel the theory presented in this book is sound, as it is the basis for understanding the need for change. Understanding the theory is fundamental to mastering new skills.

Concerns of the Physician

Every physician in practice has two major, equally important concerns. The first is for the *production* of results, whether they be eliminating the disease or ensuring that all of the activities essential for patient care have been carried out. This means supervising, often indirectly and often after the fact, anyone involved in the care provided and, of course, that includes the patients themselves. Procedures must be performed and progress reports completed. But often, and more importantly, it means conveying information and reaching a high level of comprehension and understanding with a patient in a face-to-face setting. Medicine is increasingly a job of time management and of setting priorities based on the response of those paramedical professionals you depend on to carry out your instruction-the "orders" that are a direct reflection of your leadership style. Production is also measured by patient load, diagnostic tests completed, and length of hospital stay. As medicine gets more complex and more organized, with ever more services subcontracted, hospital based, or qualified by a contract (managed care, PPO, HMO, etc.), your attention is likely to turn increasingly often to a "concern for production." Building your practice is part of this concern, but *production* can also be thought of as a shorthand term for the complexities we have come to know as "the cure.

The other major concern is for *patients,* not solely the elimination of their disease or the mending of their wounds, but a concern for them as people. Concern for the people who are the patients is evident in several ways: how the physician gathers information, listens for feedback from them, understands their expectations, makes decisions with them or on their behalf, meets their special needs, evaluates their deeper understanding, accepts their criticism, resolves conflicts with them, and motivates behavioral change. Each individual is the physician's responsibility during the patient-physician encounter, as he or she may virtually never reach out for help in any other setting, and it has been shown in numerous studies that the care provider has greatest influence on health behavioral change. Individuals may feel compelled to return to their physician repeatedly, but only for short-term medical care and often to gain temporary relief from a self-induced disease; or they can be empowered with the ability to initiate self-care, the only long-term solution to our health-care crisis. Each interaction demands imagination, innovation, and creativity. Giving patients understanding, personal responsibility, and the self-esteem needed to care for themselves is essential to achieve the highest quality required by this new medical era.

The traditional problem that has faced physicians is that neither the concern for production nor the concern for patients, as they come together in a *leadership style,* has been formally taught in medical schools or residency programs. Medical facts and clinical decisions have been enough to overwhelm students and residents and to provide the constant challenge of reeducation for the established clinician. However, for physicians ready to face the real health care crisis in this country, the need also exists to acquire leadership skills as the first step towards integrating these concerns in order to achieve true excellence in the delivery of medical care. The quality of leadership in these terms makes the critical difference, as these principles are a requirement for defining the professional relationships that we need to achieve the highest quality of care.

The Physician Grid

The way in which these two concerns interact is called a Grid strategy, demonstrated visually on the Physician Grid in Figure 1-1. This Grid is laid out on two 9-point scales, where 1 represents low, 5 is average, and 9 is high concern. The horizontal axis indicates a concern for curing the disease, building the practice, and making the ever-more-complex technology of medicine work. The vertical axis represents concern for the patient as a person. The numbers between 1, 5, and 9 indicate intermediate degrees of concern. The level of each type of concern helps to characterize the style of leadership the physician uses in everyday practice situations.

It should be easy to see that some styles help to create difficult patients while others easily meet their needs. Considering all 81 different combinations of these two concerns that are represented in a 9 X 9 point system would be an exceedingly complex task. We do not intend to analyze these multiple combinations, but rather to clarify the theories and strategies of medical practice represented by the corner and midpoint Grid positions so that you can see your own leadership style more clearly. This self-analysis is a first step toward developing the structure necessary for personal change through the expansion of your leadership abilities.

9,1

In the lower right-hand corner, the 9,1 orientation identifies a physician who is determined to find the cure, to be the ever-present expert, the all-knowing authority, with little or no concern for the patient as a human being. The patient

Figure 1-1. The Physician Grid

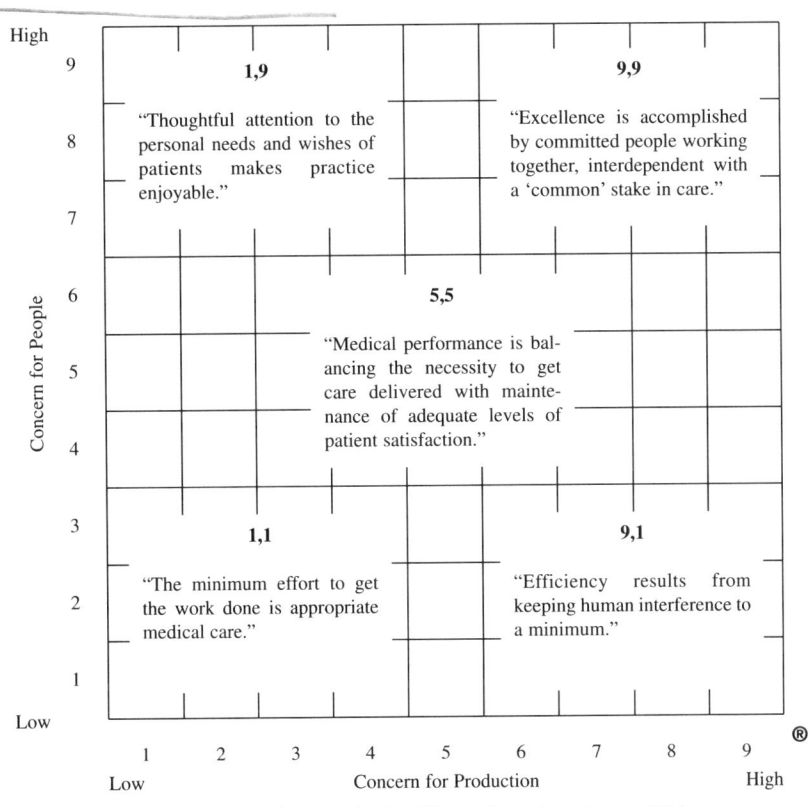

(The Grid® is a registered trademark of Scientific Methods, Inc., Austin, TX.)

is viewed as the carrier of disease and injury from which a cure may be extracted. A subject for performance, the patient is not considered capable of participating in or even understanding the complexities of the process being applied to the cure. The physician with a maximum concern for production (9) combined with a minimum concern for people (1) maximizes production by exercising power and authority. Control over other professionals, personnel, and patients themselves is achieved by dictating what each individual should do and exactly how it should be done.

Such 9,1 assumptions can result in behavior that alienates the patient and those individuals in the organization of medicine who are required to support the physician's decisions. It is an insensitive, hard-driving, hard-sell approach. During academic training, almost every physician has been exposed to clinicians like this-so bent on curing the patient and teaching the medical rules that they have become blind to the needs of those around them, to how patients feel, and to the unresolved reservations or doubts that build into a lack of trust.

This physician-patient relationship can create a win-lose battle or can result in poor patient compliance. In some cases, it leads eventually to the patient's abandoning the medical system for an unproven practice or simply falling back into unsupervised, often medically suspect, self-care and follow-up. Quality care is at that point no longer possible.

1,9

The 1,9 practice strategy is in the upper left-hand corner. Here the physician feels a minimum degree of concern for curing the patient but a maximum concern for the person behind the disease. This concern also extends to all of those colleagues and individuals required for the delivery of medical care. Making these individuals feel good is essential, even if it is at the expense of achieving the results required to cure the patient. Most of the physician's time is spent being nice, striving for a friendly relationship, often engaging in small talk as an attempt to be more socially acceptable. This physician views the cure of the patient as a byproduct of friendliness and trust, rather than as a direct consequence of ensuring excellence in medical decision making and management.

The desire to be liked may improve the physician's image, but it can be a liability when it becomes the overriding concern and the physician begins to rely on friendships for survival. Even if patients choose not to sue such a "good ol' boy," a patient who receives poor care has been grossly cheated out of the very fundamental service that is the heart of medicine. Furthermore, even a patient who is not really difficult and who personally likes the physician may not overlook flagrant errors that have resulted from inattention to the continuing education required to maintain expertise.

9+9

The paternalistic approach to leadership is embodied in a well- known physician style, best understood as a combination of 9,1 and 1,9. Called *paternalism,* it is at the very root of medicine. The paternalistic physician is not only technically expert, but also feels an overwhelming obligation to "be there" for the patient. At first glance 9+9 resembles a 9,9 orientation, but on closer examination this physician is not really attuned to the unique needs of each patient. Rather, this somewhat self-righteous banner carrier for the virtues of medicine already knows what is best for the patient and tends to make patients who "can't comply" feel guilty, while rewarding those who follow directions with praise.

This physician is a perfectionist, which is not a bad quality in medicine, but, in return for the cure, he or she expects blind loyalty from the patient. The loving "father knows best" image is familiar to all of us in the guise of Dr. Welby, but this idealized version did not let the public see the associated condescending character who says, "I know what's best for you. There, there, it will be all right." This kind of caring keeps children from harming themselves, but it is patronizing to adults. When it serves as the basis for patient care, dependency is created on one hand and frustration at not being allowed genuine participation in decision making is created on the other hand. When a poor outcome results, these patients see themselves as betrayed by the best medical knowledge available. They do not understand why the system has let them down. This physician undoubtedly feels mystified when a patient sues, because their relationship has been one of caring. It is the frustration coupled with dependency that creates the volatile situation. As a result of a poor outcome, the physician's approach is seen as wrong, and the patient's response to feeling like a fool for acting the part of a child is a lawsuit. Here again, the physician's style has actually helped to create the difficult patient and has allowed the highest quality result to slip away.

1,1

A minimum level of concern for both production and the human element is represented by the 1,1 strategy at the lower left corner of the Grid. The physician's interests in curing the patient and in the patient as a human being are both at low ebb. This physician is best characterized as "burned out," doing the minimum required to survive in practice. Minimal effort is exerted toward follow-up, accurate decision making, and any management required to provide optimal care; nor is any real attempt made to establish the type of relationship with the patient that creates trust or even understanding. The basic practice style can be summed up as "going through the motions." It is actually hard to call this individual a physician at all, but he or she has learned to survive by putting out just enough to get by, and by falling back on a legal system that guarantees the physician a right to a livelihood as long as a patient will still walk through the door.

This physician also creates difficult patients because this style destroys trust, as it addresses neither the technical nor the personal needs of the patient and is the most likely practice style to create a deterioration in quality and a poor medical outcome. High-risk medical situations, if encountered, are not met successfully; with dissatisfaction, the patient will either abandon the system or sue.

5,5

The center of the Grid depicts a 5,5 strategy, which is a "middle-of-the-road" philosophy representing half of each kind of concern. This is a common model for the physician who is established and secure. There is no hard push to grow or to continue the medical education required to achieve ever higher quality care. Concern for the patient is best described as creating a cordial atmosphere for patient interaction. The "go along to get along" attitude is revealed by conformity to the status quo.

The physician is generally well liked, telling a joke or talking about sports or the weather as a way of breaking the ice with patients and colleagues and of maintaining a friendly repartee. Underneath it all is a reliance on set routines with pat prescriptions and a rehearsed "sophistication"; all of these come through after awhile as mechanical and studied, because that is exactly what they are.

Patients easily see through this facade as the lack of personal attention is consistent, regardless of the situation or the concern of the patient. This attitude lends itself well to a clinical situation in which all patients are treated the same by all doctors. The lack of individualization that characterizes the physician-patient relationship is the reason complaints are voiced against "clinic care." Even though it falls into acceptable parameters of therapy, it is a far cry from medical excellence, but, interestingly, it is a rapidly growing practice style. Trust is threatened this time because the patients are not sure the doctor sees them and their problems as unique. This style certainly does not adapt to the needs of difficult patients and, once again, a dissatisfied patient is likely to sue.

9,9

The 9,9 strategy is in the upper right-hand corner. This depicts the model for the physician of the future. It is the style that integrates high levels of concern for both production and the human being behind the medical care that physicians provide. It is a goal-centered team approach that is designed to gain optimal results — not only through advanced technology, but also through the participation and, most importantly, the cooperation of all those directing care to patients. Patients are brought into the team as significant contributors to the overall outcome of medical care. The patients' human potential nearly always benefits from this type of approach, regardless of the final physical outcome in the management of the patients' diseases. This physician has achieved the integration of the concerns necessary for the highest quality outcome through excellence in medical care.

During the physician-patient interaction, the 9,9 concern for cure is evident through comprehensive medical knowledge coupled with the ability to relate this knowledge convincingly to the patient. The concomitant high concern for the patient as a human being is revealed through two-way communication focused on the patient's needs, expectations, level of understanding, and ability to participate in the treatment.

The 9,9 orientation reflects a deep respect for medical advancements and an understanding of the complexity inherent in delivering medical care. It also reveals a sometimes deeper concern for the patient as a fellow human being whose ill health requires the services that the committed physician continues to develop and perfect. The patient response, and the response of the entire medical team, is trust.

The Significance of Dominant Medical Practice Grid Styles In Caring For Difficult Patients

Understanding the basis of your own Grid style is the first step toward caring for the difficult patient. It also provides the cornerstones for achieving leadership excellence in medical practice regardless of your usual style. The medical-practice Grid concept rests on a set of theories about how people use their intelligence and skills in working with and through other people. When personal change is required to cope with difficult situations, this book may help you to take the often difficult first step that leads ultimately to a change in patient understanding and responsibility.

You may be able to identify your dominant Grid style without very much analysis. Characteristics that do not fit the assumptions of this dominant style may also be relatively easy to recognize. However, understanding your dominant practice style is influenced by three major conditions:

1. *Personal History*. A physician's dominant practice style, to a large degree, is rooted in personal history. We all become predisposed to one particular approach or another based on past experience, good and bad outcomes, and "learning the hard way." Although Grid style is not the same as personality, it is a reflection of what we assume about ourselves and about others as we try to lead them and is thus related to our natural technique of leading others in every walk of life.

2. *Organization*. Medical-practice behavior is being increasingly influenced by organizations and the need to belong in this new era. At one time, physicians simply joined their licensing organization or the fraternities of the American Medical Association or subspecialty organizations. Rules and requirements were minimal. Physicians were left largely to private practice, organizing their own office structures, and simply being obligated to meet their professional code of ethics and the privilege delineations for practice at a particular hospital. Now we have entered an era of PHOs, HMOs, and "provider-at-risk" care. Hospital regulations demand new sets of rules and requirements that strictly define interactions of paramedical personnel with physicians. Using DRGs, actual practice patterns are being evaluated in the form of audits that review the number of days per diagnosis. Physicians are

being screened for participation in payor panels on the basis of the cost-benefit ratio of laboratory tests ordered as well as outcome data from computerized quality assurance assessment programs. Insurance companies are requiring second opinions and outpatient management rather than hospitalization for certain diagnoses. Leadership style is beginning to reflect fewer personal assumptions and more of the assumptions directed to achieving organization results. The expression, *The right way to manage a case,* has already moved from personal preference to the courts of medical-legal litigation, quality assurance professionals, panels of peer review organizations, and executive boards of "organized medicine." It is becoming increasingly more difficult to ignore these influences on your ability to consistently maintain a practice style that can achieve medical excellence, even when faced with downsized facilities, let alone a crisis or the difficult patient's response to stress.

3. *Values.* The dominant Grid practice style is also affected by assumptions the physician makes on the basis of his or her values, beliefs, or ideals. Some are led into medicine because of the desire to be of service, the prestige of being a doctor, or the financial gain. Still others may enter because of fascination with the high-tech world of medicine. A desire to please parents may motivate others. Each of these reasons reflects different personal values that influence the kind of practice style that becomes characteristic of a particular physician. A personal belief system influences attitudes about the way patients should be treated and the way peers and paramedical personnel need to function in order to ensure high-quality medical care. It is this influence that reminds us of the purpose of medicine in an era that is emphasizing techniques of mere survival. As much as in any profession, values are a pivotal point in establishing the relationships with human beings that are essential to medical practice. The purpose of medicine is the relief of pain and suffering, and the creation of optimal human potential through improving the quality and increasing the longevity of life. These very goals are the result of what we deem to be important as human beings.

The Shift From Dominant to Back-up Grid Styles

The physician's Grid style may be consistent over a range of situations. A physician can maintain the same Grid style when interviewing, teaching, practicing, making decisions, supporting families, keeping confidential information, organizing vast quantities of both personal and technical information, and finally managing whatever medical team is involved in the care of a patient. However, a physician can also shift Grid styles depending upon stress, the kind of stress that occurs typically when faced with a crisis, a difficult patient, or both. The reason that a dominant set of Grid assumptions can be reconciled with leadership styles that shift and change is that most of us have a dominant Grid style backed up by a second, third, or even fourth style applied to the various situations that we face on a day-to-day basis.

It is important to remember that the style or styles employed by physicians as they work can be complex. The dominant or most characteristic style is the one most central to understanding how a physician usually conducts his or her practice; however, a back-up style, that which is used next most commonly, is employed when the dominant style becomes difficult or even impossible to apply appropriately. We commonly see a back-up style emerge under pressure or to deal with situations in which the dominant Grid style has already failed to resolve conflict. A great array of dominant-back-up combinations contributes to making each person a unique practitioner, as we will see in Chapter 3.

Benefits and Limitations of the Grid Approach

Benefits

The Grid framework, which permits comparison of similarities and differences in leadership styles, serves as a conceptual model on which to build leadership and, ultimately, the medical excellence that it ensures. This leadership is what caring for difficult patients is all about. Consequences as they directly affect productivity, creativity, patient satisfaction, and physician career success can be easily evaluated using this model. The approach is self-directed, allowing you to draw your own conclusions based on your perception of what constitutes effective leadership.

Empirical assessment of the validity of the 9,9 orientation in comparison with others has been developed in over 50 years of research on leadership style and operational consequences in various fields of endeavor. The Grid framework has been independently assessed for its conceptual validity and has been found to meet the highest standards for conceptual logic. The 9,9 orientation is a scientifically derived theory and, therefore, a logical, reproducible structure that meets the discriminating demands of the physician.

The Grid provides a common language for discussing the goals of clinical practice improvement efforts, as well as issues of leadership, practice management, and patient understanding. It permits physicians and paramedical personnel to discuss and agree among themselves on the role of leadership in the interactions of a well-functioning medical team. In this same context, the Grid provides a basic model for developing an organized medical team characterized not only by effective leadership, but also by sound participation-based teamwork throughout its membership. This method can be used constructively by anyone of any technical background who is part of the team, regardless of his or her level of experience. Success in the new era of medicine demands that the physician face a variety of situations in which he or she must achieve results with and through people.

The pressures of new organizations in medicine can be met using the Grid approach, which is applicable to any size group (from 5 to 5,000 persons) in which sound leadership is required. This approach is pertinent at every level of nurse interaction, in office staff organization, and in supervising the medical team. It can be used as a technique to better understand the part a patient plays as a member of the various teams now required to deliver medical care.

The Grid system is, more importantly, a tool that can be used to evaluate patients, to improve their understanding of medical decision making, and to lead them toward a 9,9 response to medical advice.

Medical practice has evolved to a point where patient education and shared decision making are requirements, and the Grid can serve as the structure to encourage individualizing information, ensuring understanding, and providing true informed consent.

Finally, the Grid framework has an application to family life, child rearing, and volunteer activities in communities where physicians continue to be leaders and to find themselves placed in positions of responsibility with other people.

Limitations

Critics of this type of approach to clinical leadership is a part of coping with difficult situations or difficult patients. They have already given up and chosen to concentrate on enforced expert standards and defense trial strategies. Or if they agree that leadership is a key, they feel that it is a natural ability and that you either have it or you do not. They say, therefore, that it cannot be taught; yet the very basis of growth for a medical student is a lesson in leadership. The real problem is that the lesson has not gone far enough.

Others think that you can learn to be a leader but that "you can't teach an old dog new tricks," or that it is possible to teach the highly motivated, but everyone else is a lost cause. These skeptics state that leadership does not have a place in continuing medical education. Accepting either of these propositions is to say that physicians are somehow less bright or less motivated than the many professionals who have undertaken similar programs with great success. These critics of training programs deny that physicians can learn to be more effective, yet the concept that effectiveness is teachable is at the heart of medical education.

These value-based beliefs negate the possibilities of human learning and rest on false assumptions. It is as practical to learn to lead effectively as it is to learn to tie surgical knots or, for that matter, to perfect any other applied skill. The time required to learn effective leadership skills is a fraction of the time taken to learn even one of the subdisciplines of medicine and is the one area of education that can impact the quality of care provided by *all* physicians, regardless of their specialty.

Chapter Two

THE GRID MIRROR

Because the character of physician leadership is a significant factor in being able to care for difficult patients, not to mention professional success or failure, this book focuses on leadership by comparing that which is effective with that which *is not*. Our goal is to answer fundamental questions about how to exercise your leadership in caring for patients in all types of difficult situations. You will learn about behaviors that limit your effectiveness and about those that are sound. The benefits to be gained include strengthening your contribution to the field of medicine and increasing the likelihood of achieving high-quality outcomes, as well as ensuring a successful and rewarding career in medical practice.

This book is intended to help you be more objective in discovering how to positively impact your quality outcomes profile, as well as to prevent unfounded claims of poor care by increasing your own effectiveness. It therefore must guide you in being more self-analytical about your present ways of practicing medicine. What you are about to study is your leadership style. It is this initial step that allows a needed perspective for all that follows.

Elements of Leadership

Leadership is a complex process. However, six main elements, each a step in the progression of patient care, can be isolated and examined. All six of these elements — *communication, acquiring knowledge, decision making, conflict resolution, initiative,* and *critique and feedback* — are vital to effective leadership, because none can compensate for the lack or overabundance of any other, and each impacts on the others.

The six elements of leadership are briefly described in the following sections. Within each section are six statements that characterize different leadership approaches. You will notice that all of the A statements reflect the same leadership approach, as do all the B through F statements.

At this point, it may be worthwhile for you to take a quick look at yourself as a physician. This can enable you to cut beneath the surface and to see how the remaining material in the book may alter your relationships with patients. Read the sentences beneath each element, considering each as a possible description of yourself. Put a 6 beside the sentence that you think is most like you. Then continue ranking the other sentences from 5 to 1. A 1 should be placed next to the sentence that is least characteristic of you. There can be no ties. These statements provide benchmarks for recognizing leadership as a process of people working together to achieve objectives.

Communication

Communication is the basis for the physician-patient interaction during the delivery of medical care. A physician may have strong convictions but think it risky to take a stand. Alternatively, the physician may not advocate a position because of low or nonexistent convictions. The physician also may embrace a point of view simply to oppose someone or to win an argument.

A_____ I keep my own counsel but respond when asked. I avoid taking sides by not revealing my opinions, attitudes, and ideas.

B_____ I embrace opinions, attitudes, and ideas of patients, even though I have reservations.

C_____ I express opinions, attitudes, and ideas in a tentative way and try to meet patients halfway.

D_____ I stand up for my opinions, attitudes, and ideas, even if it means rejecting the patients' views.

E_____ I maintain strong convictions but permit patients to express their ideas so that I can help them think more objectively.

F_____ I feel it is important to express my concerns and convictions. I respond to ideas sounder than my own by changing my mind.

Acquiring Knowledge

Inquiry is the aspect of communication that permits a physician to uncover facts and to gather data from patients as well as other information sources that impact medical care. The quality of inquiry may range from ignoring the need for inquiry to being keenly interested in learning as much as possible.

A_____ I go along with facts, beliefs, and positions given to me.

B_____ I look for facts, beliefs, and positions that suggest all is well. For the sake of harmony, I am not inclined to challenge patients.

C_____ I take things more or less at face value and check facts, beliefs, and positions only when obvious discrepancies appear.

D_____ I investigate facts, beliefs, and positions so that I am in control of any situation and to assure myself that patients are not making mistakes.

E_____ I double-check what patients tell me and compliment them when I am able to verify their compliance.

F_____I search for and validate information. I invite and listen for opinions, attitudes, and ideas different from my own.I continuously reevaluate my own and patients' facts, beliefs, and positions for soundness.

Decision Making

It is through decision making that leadership impacts performance and, ultimately, the quality of medical care. It may involve solo decision making, in which the physician alone is the ultimate decision maker, or a team of staff, patients, and colleagues, through which all available resources are brought to bear on making decisions.

A_____ I let others make decisions or come to terms with whatever happens.

B_____ I search for decisions that maintain good relations and encourage patients to make decisions when possible.

C_____ I search for workable decisions that patients accept.

D_____ I insist on making decisions and am rarely influenced by others.

E_____ I have the final say and make a sincere effort to see that my decisions are accepted.

F_____ I place high value on arriving at sound decisions. I seek understanding and agreement.

Initiative

Initiative, an outgrowth of decision making, is exercised whenever effort is concentrated on a specific activity: to start something that was not going on before, to stop something that was occurring, or to shift the direction and character of effort. A physician may take initiative or may avoid it even when patients expect action.

A_____ I put out enough to get by.

B_____ I initiate actions that help and support patients.

C_____ I seek to maintain a steady pace.

D_____ I drive myself and my patients.

E_____ I stress loyalty and extend appreciation to those patients who follow my directives.

F_____ I exert vigorous effort and patients join in enthusiastically.

Conflict Resolution

When patients have different points of view and express them, disagreements are inevitable. Conflict can be either disruptive and destructive or creative and constructive, depending on how it is handled. A physician who can face conflict with patients and resolve it to their mutual understanding evokes respect. The inability to cope with conflict constructively leads to disrespect, even to increased hostility and antagonism.

A_____ I remain neutral or seek to stay out of conflict.

B_____ I avoid generating conflict, but when it appears I try to soothe feelings to keep patients satisfied.

C_____ When conflict arises, I try to find a reasonable position that patients find suitable.

D_____ When conflict arises, I try to cut it off or win my position.

E_____ When conflict arises, I terminate it but thank the patients for expressing their views.

F_____ When conflict arises, I seek out reasons for it in order to resolve underlying causes.

Critique and Feedback

Critique and feedback constitute a process of stepping away from or interrupting an activity to study it, to consider alternative possibilities for improving performance, and to anticipate and avoid any activities that have adverse consequences. A physician may or may not consider day-to-day practice as a basis for learning and may or may not share reactions with others through feedback. Without such learning, medical excellence is unlikely to be achieved. Critique and feedback provide the basis for learning from experience so as to work more effectively with patients through the medical team.

A_____ I avoid giving feedback.

B_____ I give encouragement and offer praise when patients comply, but avoid giving negative feedback.

C_____ I give informal or indirect feedback regarding suggestions for improvement.

D_____ I pinpoint weaknesses or failure to comply.

E_____ I give patients feedback and expect them to accept it because it is for their own good.

F_____ I encourage two-way feedback to strengthen the physician-patient relationship.

Having completed the self-assessment, you may or may not see a pattern in your practice style. The statements in each area of leadership characterize particular Grid styles and rest on certain *assumptions* about how to achieve the best medical outcome while meeting the patients' needs. The way in which assumptions guide behavior is discussed in the following section.

How Assumptions Guide Behavior

Whether you recognize them or not, assumptions are at the center of your most comfortable practice strategy. Whenever physicians approach a situation, they appraise it subjectively. This appraisal includes assumptions about what is true or reliable. Objective reality and the subjective appraisal of it can be close together or far apart. Assumptions, then, are what give your style of practice its unique character — either contributing to its success in a variety of situations or limiting its effectiveness with difficult patients.

Many examples illustrate how assumptions shape behavior. Assumptions about illness, for example, lead to treatment by magic in one culture and to cure through medicine in another. Some cultures assume that dictatorship is the way to organize the activities of people. The belief of others is that constitutional democracy or limited monarchy is best. The point for our work is that assumptions shape our relationships with our patients and our ways of practicing medicine. When an assumption we make is also being made by those around us, for practical purposes it becomes an absolute not to be questioned. Other possible assumptions are ignored. The "absolute" eliminates courses of action that are inconsistent with those assumptions and blinds everyone to options that might produce sounder medical care.

Physicians seldom verbalize their assumptions, but they do act on them. The concept that all assumptions are "equal but different" has appeal in that it permits leaders from many walks of life to avoid making a choice, but not all assumptions are equal as a basis for exercising effective medical care. For the physician, making choices is a necessity, and the choice of assumptions becomes an important issue to consider, because some assumptions lead to good outcomes and others lead to poor ones.

A comprehensive theory of physician leadership is possible because only a limited number of assumptions about how to achieve performance with and through others is available. It is important to understand our own assumptions because they operate silently and their central role in controlling our behavior is likely to be unseen. Reducing this self-blindness is one purpose of the Grid. Understanding our assumptions about leadership can help us to see the impact of our behavior on the efforts of those with whom we work and on our patients. Awareness of just what those assumptions are is the first step to change.

Assumptions Can Be Changed

Sometimes we explain something we did by saying, "I assumed that..." or "...that assumption didn't work." Far more often, we are completely unaware of the assumptions that underlie our conduct. We are as baffled about why we do things as others are in trying to explain our actions. Without new insights to challenge our assumptions, we have difficulty identifying them. With new experiences and feedback from others regarding our actions, assumptions can be reexamined and change becomes possible.

The Grid helps us examine assumptions about leadership and how they apply to medical care. Once we become aware of the depth and character of our assumptions, we can identify the positive and negative consequences of actions based on them. We can consider alternative assumptions that may provide a sounder basis for medical practice, and by applying these assumptions in a variety of difficult situations, we can make them characteristic of our unique style as physicians.

Summary

By using Grid theory to identify assumptions that underlie all of patient care, physicians can see themselves and others more objectively, communicate more clearly, understand where their disagreements come from, learn how to change themselves, and help even the most difficult patients undergoing medical care to move toward a more satisfying experience and also ensure the highest quality outcome. The more skilled a physician becomes in using a sound theory of leadership, the more capable that physician is of reducing frustration, resentment, and other negative emotions that epitomize the experience with difficult patients and all patients faced with less-than-perfect outcomes. The shift away from these feelings toward enthusiasm and understanding is the result of sound leadership and is the reward for making the efforts to bring about needed change.

Chapter Three

THE IMPORTANCE OF THE PATIENT GRID TO PHYSICIAN-PATIENT INTERACTION

Once you have detailed exactly what your assumptions are, you are ready to address the other individual in the physician-patient interaction. As you can imagine, the patient also has a set of assumptions. Many times these are not well understood by the patient, especially at a time of crisis, yet they dramatically affect the manner in which he or she approaches you as a physician. Difficult patients suddenly emerge under stress, or they are obvious from the start; but their assumptions and, in a way, their leadership style provide landmarks that you can learn to recognize. Your own strategies for patient care can be developed in the light of the assumptions and approaches that your patient brings to the physician-patient interaction.

The Patient Grid

Patients, similar to physicians, enter into the patient-physician interaction with two concerns. One is the concern for getting well — for receiving the service of the physician. This is represented by the horizontal axis of the Patient Grid, Figure 3-1. The second, represented on the vertical axis, indicates the degree of concern the patients have for you, the physician. This attitude is critical, as you are the individual to whom they have chosen to entrust their bodies, their fears, and their expectations. In addition, like physicians, each patient has his or her own strategy and tactics that guide behavior within the entire medical health care complex. Understanding the patient's perspective is critical in determining who the difficult patients are, so that you can begin to meet their needs.

9,1

Patients who are 9,1 oriented have maximum concern for getting the best

Figure 3-1. The Patient Grid.

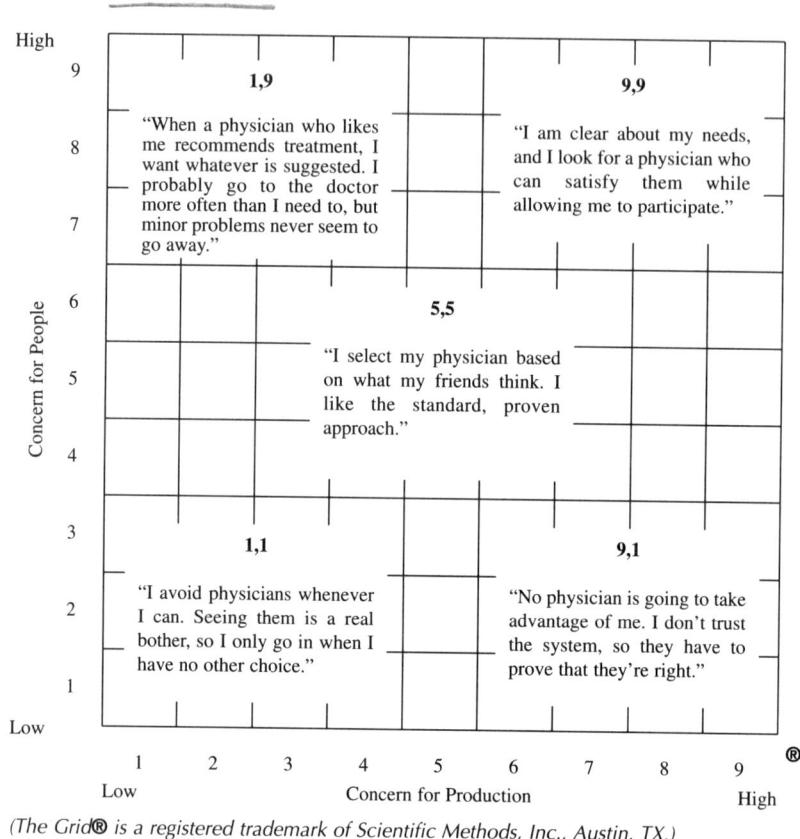

(The Grid® is a registered trademark of Scientific Methods, Inc., Austin, TX.)

treatment, coupled with almost no concern for you as the physician. These patients simply do not trust the medical complex or the physician as the provider of care. They feel that the only option is to take control, rejecting your care if there is any doubt about their getting exactly the treatment they think they need. They fear that if they do not take this position, you will take advantage of them against their will. Their approach is likely to be pessimistic, distrusting, and aggressive. They clearly doubt that you can meet their needs, and they attempt to provoke you into proving yourself and the treatment you have recommended. With an inadequate knowledge base, they often focus on the controversies being discussed in the media and expect you to explain these controversies to their satisfaction.

Such patients may only feel good about the therapy you describe if convinced that they got the best of you, which was, indeed, their original objective. You are up against closed minds and strong convictions. A relationship with a 9,1-oriented patient can turn into a battle, with the result that no medical care is delivered, even though the treatment you recommend could have satisfied the real medical needs of the individual. Alternatively, the patients may "win" and convince you to give them what they came for, even though it is not actually what is needed. The physician, of course, is blamed for the outcomes in both situations. The problems stem from the patients' high concern for control in purchasing your services, with no understanding or regard for your role as physician and care provider — or human being, for that matter.

1,9

Patients who are 1,9 oriented have a low concern for the medical therapy you recommend, coupled with a high human concern for you as the physician, leaving no doubt about the pleasure derived from the opportunity to visit you for care. By revealing a lack of knowledge about personal health or the disease involved, the patients give the physician something to talk about. Suggestions are readily accepted, without requesting proof or even the reassurance of statistics that demonstrate the appropriateness of treatment. So as not to offend you, their response to the prescription or therapy is affirmative head shakes and pleased, often exaggerated, enthusiasm. In the physician's presence, these patients are suggestible and easily influenced. However, upon returning to a social environment critical of physicians, they may easily become disenchanted, particularly if the treatment results in a poor outcome.

These 1,9-oriented patients seek services from a physician whom they like and who accepts them as "good" patients. Such patients are generally well liked by the physician, as "understanding the importance of my advice." They are susceptible to flattery and approval, and are particularly responsive to the physician who has made the effort to memorize birth dates, children's names, and special interests. Making these individuals feel appreciated results in dedicated, devoted patients who cannot say "no," for to do so would be to reject the physician. Nevertheless, purchasing such services may be financially unwise and medically unnecessary; ultimately, it may even lead to awkward situations created by surgery that was not indicated. These patients are often overlooked as difficult patients, but with a poor outcome they often feel that they have been taken advantage of.

1,1

Patients who are 1,1 oriented have a low concern for their own health and cure as well as a low concern for the physician, and they quickly communicate their lack of interest. A typical attitude is "Physicians are always trying to tell you what's good for you, so I just avoid them." Treatment of such patients is made increasingly difficult because they may come to you not out of personal interest in their own health, but because they are pressured to do so by others. When these patients become ill, requiring hospitalization or other treatment, physician-patient interactions inevitably occur. These patients are uninterested in this interaction because the physician's service is not really wanted and has been turned to only as a last resort to escape the pressure and pain of the illness that has befallen them. Their indifference places the full weight on the physician to make all medical decisions regarding the patient's case and to provide the momentum for patient compliance.

The mind-set of these patients is to find the path of least resistance while just barely staying out of hot water. These patients are typified by individuals who abuse their health through habits such as smoking, alcohol, drug abuse, and overeating. They are health burnouts trying to stall for more time to continue their ill behavior by avoiding the input of a physician who must tell them that they are killing themselves. When they are forced to see you, their lack of concern for you, the physician, is obvious. They simply perceive you as someone willing to shift their responsibility to your shoulders. The physician who accepts this responsibility must be aware of the contract that has just been entered into. Documentation of this inadequate relationship may be the only way to cope with these truly hard cases.

5,5

Patients who take a middle position, expecting to be treated professionally in a give-and-take manner and responding with appropriate politeness in the physician-patient interaction, are in the 5,5 orientation. Such patients do not want to be challenged to think deeply, but desire solutions that sound familiar or that have been accepted with confidence by others in their peer group; they feel uncomfortable receiving any care other than that which is standard and routine. The physician's prestige and confidence may move a 5,5-oriented patient toward acceptance of a given therapy as long as the prescription does not violate the conventional thinking of their peers. These patients also may accept therapy based on name dropping or tidbits they have heard about past patients who were satisfied with their treatment.

New therapies can be expected to raise objections, primarily because these patients fear being made to look foolish: "What will other people think if I take this advice?" The difficulty with 5,5-oriented patients is that the original complaint may have no bearing on whether the patients accept or reject the recommended cure. Favorable response to the treatment plan very often will depend on the fad being followed this year and the social group to which the patients belong. At the same time, patients worry about the existence of better treatments, unless the medical therapy in question has a recognized and established degree of sophistication and efficacy.

9,9

As you review strategies that help you cope with problem patients, it soon becomes clear that your goal is to create 9,9-oriented patients. These patients feel deeply about making sound decisions with respect to recommended medical advice, while maintaining a high concern for you, the physician. They are accustomed to thinking and analyzing in a factually based, straightforward manner and respect you when you deal with symptoms or complaints in these terms. When the physician is not communicating well, 9,9-oriented patients are prepared to exercise personal leadership skills and redirect the discussion to a problem-solving level. They actually perceive physicians as real human beings with personal limitations and are unwilling to accept advice or purchase services on the basis of either partial knowledge or an unsound relationship between physician and patient.

The 9,9-oriented patients assess their "real needs," at least in general terms if not in medical specifics, before approaching a physician. Such patients respond favorably when the physician encourages two-way communication about the situation and how well the medical advice integrates with the patients' life requirements. By fully understanding the impact, risks, and benefits of pertinent therapies, these patients can participate in reaching sound and realistic decisions. At this point, the patients are in a position to purchase services from the physician, convinced that their mutual decision is a good one. Both patients and the physician can stand by the medical plan as sound, regardless of the outcome, shifting only when contraindications or new evidence suggests that a different plan should be introduced. This patient creates the most likely route to consistently high-quality outcomes.

The Medical Practice Grids As A Key to Physician-Patient Interaction

These five basic Patient Grid positions are only relative; the full possibility of combinations is 81, just as with the Physician Grid. Using these fundamental positions, however, aids us in becoming aware of the potential for interactions between the physician and patient. At the core of medical excellence is the leadership ability of physicians to understand these interactions and how they are influenced by assumptions that patients and physicians bring to the relationship.

The Use of Dominant and Back-up Grid Styles

By limiting our discussion to 11 major medical-practice Grid styles-six that relate to the physician and five that apply to patients — the possible combinations are not too difficult to understand and use in examining physician-patient interactions. As soon as the underlying motivations of the physician and patient become clear, the physician is well on the way toward enhancing even the most trying physician-patient relationships and experiencing the full potential of medical leadership. Back-ups complicate the picture, yet it is important for a physician to understand how patients bring about a shift from dominant to back-up Grid styles.

Although medical practice can be enhanced by the application of sound behavioral science principles alone, the art of medicine always depends to some degree on the physician's ability to sense emotional color and personal and patient bias. The nuances of innumerable combinations of stress within the patient environment must be understood so that the patient can be creatively motivated toward a good medical outcome. The specific physician-patient interactions that follow in the chapters on dominant Grid styles will make this job somewhat easier.

Before we go on, let us look at a few examples. A physician who normally practices in a 9,9 style may meet continued resistance from a patient who is unwilling to communicate in a problem-solving way. If the patient is a fighter, the physician may be lured into the 9,1 style. The physician might have been better off shifting to a 5,5 approach, negotiating for a compromise so that some of the medical care required could be provided without disrupting the patient's life style excessively. As another example, a physician might begin a meeting with a patient in a friendly and casual way, but because of an emergency, quickly move to a 9,1 approach in order to address the medical situation. Even though the beginning might have been 1,9 in character, the 9,1 back-up approach is drawn upon in a crisis so often that it is very close to the dominant style. In this case, the physician takes control of the situation without utilizing the resources of those who may be best able to contribute to a solution.

To really understand a physician's dominant and back-up approaches, you must observe behavior over time and over a range of situations. Some physicians shift frequently under less stress than others. Learning to control these unwanted shifts is a major part of the work that lies ahead.

Here is another example. A physician who usually approaches patients from a 9,1 orientation, pressing hard for results and strict obedience, may become burned out from a personal crisis, from slow advancement in an academic setting, or from the first lawsuit and, as a consequence, may become a victim who sinks into a 1,1 state of resignation. If this particular physician had had a different set of back-up assumptions that could have been used to reevaluate the situation and to formulate a plan, better medical care might have resulted, and greater career satisfaction certainly would have been ensured. The great variety of dominant-back-up behavioral combinations seen within the many situations in which physicians and patients interact is what makes the field of medicine such a fascinating, rewarding, and truly challenging profession.

The significant complexities of relationships between physicians and their patients are examined in detail in later chapters, but one major point can be made: Every indication is that the physician's Grid strategy is more important than the patient's with respect to successful communication and the quality of the medical outcome. The physician tends to set the climate of the patient-physician relationship, which encourages the patient to respond in kind, possibly moving easily from a dominant style into the desired 9,9-oriented back-up set of assumptions so that good medical care can be ensured. Just as certainly, another physician's initiative (9,1; 1,9; 9+9; 1,1; or 5,5) can create a climate that starts the physician-patient relationship moving in a downward spiral. What this means is that *the physician is in the position to exercise leadership* and therefore has the responsibility to guide the patient to sound decisions, the best possible outcome, and an understanding of the ever more complex decisions that define medical care. It is this leadership that creates lasting patient-physician relationships, valid communication, the trust required for mutual respect, and ultimately self-care.

Highly advanced technical equipment, modern and well-designed hospitals, and highly educated personnel account for little or nothing if leadership is ineffectively exercised to take advantage of the skills and sophistication currently expected in medicine. When the total picture of medical care comes together, leadership is clearly the key that facilitates the conversion of the tremendous resources available into effective, high-quality medical care.

Chapter Four

9,1 MEDICAL CARE: NOT ALWAYS RIGHT, BUT NEVER IN DOUBT

Dr. Gray led his troop of residents around the mop and bucket that had been left standing outside Mrs. Thomas' room, thinking to himself, "Someone will hear about this. The professionalism of a hospital is reflected by its employees and the manner in which the smallest job is done." Dr. Gray was on edge; he was late; the new clinical policies were forcing him to see an increased volume of patients in addition to those referred to him from around the country for his highly recognized surgical skills. He now had to add the clinical obligation to his already pressing academic assignments in order to generate income for the hospital. It was the new strategy to help pay his and other staff members' salaries. To top it off, he had just come from the business meeting where Dr. Allen, the newest member of the staff, had had the gall to question the referral service Dr. Gray had organized. It was Dr. Allen's opinion that Dr. Gray was the busiest physician on the staff as a "benefit" of being the head of the department. Dr. Gray chuckled to himself as he surveyed the unfinished janitorial task and remembered how he had mopped the floor with the inexperienced and arrogant doctor.

"Well, Dr. Allen, since you are such an authority on surgical care and who should be performing procedures at this hospital, explain to me how you could justify any change. Certainly you wouldn't suggest increasing your own patient load. As chairman of the department, it is my responsibility to keep tabs on you new physicians. Considering that you have the highest surgical complication rate, despite a relatively light surgical schedule, I am rather surprised that you would be so presumptuous as to force your opinion on this group."

Dr. Gray was clearly one of the most skilled surgeons and intelligent academicians to have graced the halls of University Hospital. The room was silent. There was an air of respect and something else — not quite fear, but more accurately a resentment sense they all shared that the old pro would have come down on them just as hard if they had been as naive as Dr. Allen, believing that the responsibility of clinical staffing should be shared more equitably. Dr. Gray had been the head of the department for nearly 20 years. His reputation spoke for itself. Anybody who had been on staff for long knew of the volatile temper and inability to tolerate incompetence that were second only to his extraordinary skills with the scalpel.

Displaying a sense of control and power that extended beyond what would be expected from his authority alone, Dr. Gray dramatically moved his group of eager residents into Room 217. Mrs. Keating was sitting up in bed, seemingly prepared for the onslaught known as teaching rounds. The only member of the group who really knew the patient was the intern who had admitted Mrs. Keating on her first night in the hospital. With him, she had shared some of her personal trials of having had a radical mastectomy for carcinoma of the breast 10 years earlier. Of course, the patient also knew Dr. Gray. Money was no object to Mrs. Keating, the author of several popular children's books and a well-known lecturer in the area of child development. She wanted the best and Dr. Gray had come highly recommended to her.

The chairman was in his finest form on rounds, describing the complications of surgery that he easily avoided through his skilled handling of situations. He focused particularly on the advantages of a modified mastectomy over the radical mastectomy Mrs. Keating had undergone before. He moved to the bedside, shaking Mrs. Keating's hand, asking her how she felt. Seeing a nod and the beginning of a smile, he was satisfied that all was well with her.

"It's amazing how far we have come in medical practice today. Only 10 years ago, this woman received a radical mastectomy, completely removing the pectoralis major muscle and leaving her chest wall exposed with limitations to the arm. Notice the edema of the left arm compared to the right. With the procedure we have just performed, we were able to salvage the muscle, thus ensuring that this patient will have full use of her extremity and none of the unsightly lymphedema which she has suffered through for 10 years, here, on her left side." He then reached for the covers, smiled reassuringly at the patient, and pulled the blanket down, just exposing the area of surgery as well as the previously operated on left rib cage. There were no breasts. One of the residents gasped slightly and quickly cleared his throat to cover his discomfort.

"It's rare that you have the opportunity to see the radical mastectomy side by side with the new modified approach that was developed in this hospital. Here you have possibly one of the best examples you will ever see of the real progress we have made in treatment of carcinoma of the breast," he said, gesturing at the patient's deformed chest. He then turned and lifted the sheet back in place, nodding a proud but understanding approval to the patient.

Mrs. Keating was expressionless, showing neither anger nor hurt, but expressionless just the same. Dr. Gray had come to recognize this response as postoperative lethargy, sedation from pain medications, and an understandable mild depression resulting from the experience of surgery. He thanked Mrs. Keating and gathered his flock to leave the room. All of the residents had listened attentively, knowing that every word he had said was true, and imagining the challenges of technical perfection that lay ahead of them as they continued their training in an effort to at least come close to the skills demonstrated by the old master.

Only the intern noticed the reflection of light coming from the corner of Mrs. Keating's eye as a tear fought its way through the emotional control that is part of the trade of an experienced writer and speaker. He reached out his hand as the others left the room. She gripped it surprisingly hard, because she knew that he understood what that experience had cost her. And then she could no longer withhold her tears. The room was empty, except for the caring young man she had already grown to like. She had no words for him, and he knew that if he stayed any longer, it would be his tears that would have to be restrained.

Dr. Gray, with his long coat flowing behind him, moved rapidly down the hallway toward the nurses' station, where he demanded to see the head nurse. "Mrs. Brown, what the hell is going on on this floor! Look at that hallway! How can we pretend to deliver the best medical care possible when we can't even keep the hallways clean?"

Mrs. Brown immediately turned to a staff nurse, "What's the meaning of this garbage in the hallway? If the custodial can't do the job, then it becomes your responsibility to put things in order. That is your room, isn't it? Find out what's going on. Now." She turned back to Dr. Gray, "I'm terribly sorry, Dr. Gray. This shouldn't have happened and won't happen again. I'll see to that."

Without a reply, Dr. Gray turned, steaming down the hallway to the next patient's room, all the while becoming a little more on edge, thinking of the increased patient load, the new group of residents to start in the spring, the parking problem, and the staff's inability to even keep the hallways cleared. Most of all, he lamented the general decline of what had once been a proud and powerful profession, admired by a society that now looked for every chance to cry malpractice and to dethrone those personally responsible for saving lives and creating the highest quality of medical care the world had ever known. It seemed incredible and completely unfair. The public and patients would never know what it took to be a doctor; because of that, they would never give him the respect and gratitude that were his due.

General Characteristics of the 9,1-Orientation to Medicine

The 9,1 Grid style is shown in the lower right-hand corner of the Grid, where a high degree of concern for technical excellence is coupled with a low concern for people. Physicians practicing in this style have a tremendous sense of strength and power, reinforced by the great admiration held for them as physicians. Submitting to nothing and no one, and expecting obedience and a high level of performance from staff and patients epitomize physicians who have this practice style. They are hard working and willing to expend extraordinary amounts of time and effort grappling with the ever more technical problems related to curing the patient and eliminating the disease.

Motivation

These physicians are motivated by a drive to master the tremendous volume of information as well as the procedures required to remain medically expert. Their positive motivation is to control every detail of the medical practice. This includes the patient, the medical team, and the administrative staff, inasmuch as independence of thought or judgment can interfere with efficiency, accuracy, and perfection. 9,1-oriented physicians are exacting taskmasters. When others express opinions, their ideas are likely to be disregarded because these physicians, although not always right, are rarely in doubt. Being busy is all the indication necessary to reassure them that their way — "the only way" — is optimal medicine. Signing every order, double-checking the responsibilities of the paramedical personnel, and demanding appropriate records from nurses and updates on policy from administration are all ways of acquiring and maintaining control over others. However, these demands may actually be self-defeating, resulting in failure rather than mastery and domination.

The fear of failure negatively motivates the 9,1-oriented physician. Not being right hints of incompetence or malpractice. An action that is questioned by a strong-willed nurse, administrator or, even worse, a strong-willed patient is a direct challenge to clinical expertise; and when faced by a challenge, the physician applies the persistence necessary to prevail.

The technical aspects of medical care can actually flourish under such highly motivated individuals, but the need to control keeps 9,1-oriented physicians detached from the true needs and feelings of their patients and coworkers. No one questions their dedication to, or reverence for, their role as physicians; but upholding their own positions and decisions can become more important than maintaining trust based on objectivity and mutual respect. 9,1 motivations go beyond seeking to accumulate money, wealth, or other external trappings of power. Control is what is important, and domination is the measure of power in the network of relationships in which the physician is so central.

The 9,1-Oriented Physician-Patient Relationship

Providing Patient Care

To illustrate how the 9,1 Grid style elements affect the quality of patient care and create the problems that may be encountered, the six aspects of 9,1-oriented medical practice need to be examined.

Communication. 9,1 communication tends to be one way. Absolute statements are a tip-off to this attitude. Words such as *impossible, never, always,* or *everyone* are often used. Positions are viewed as either right or wrong, leaving no room for argument. Tentativeness is regarded as a sign of weakness; certainty a sign of strength. Discussion is not invited.

The physician typically is not listening for understanding but is mentally rehearsing the next point while someone else is speaking. Interrupting the opponent, whether it be patient, peer, or medical staff, to make a point is a common practice, especially if the conversation is headed in a direction that does not support the viewpoint of the physician.

Eventually the physician may be seen as closed minded, and colleagues, as well as staff and even patients, may stop presenting their positions, saying "What's the use? Why bother?"

Establishing patient expectations. One of the best methods of establishing expectations is to prevent misconceptions in the first place. The 9,1-oriented physician's approach is to communicate precisely what needs to be done in a manner designed to be convincing. Medical training programs present students with a method to use in this kind of communication. Instructions are given one step at a time, in the belief that this reduces the likelihood of confusion or error. By limiting instructions to what, where, when, and how the physician intends to proceed, the question "why" is reduced in importance. When the physician asks, "Do you understand?" the patients are expected to answer "yes," but it is a yes as to what is to happen, not why. Patients respond "yes" to a 9,1-oriented physician's query, even on those occasions when they do not understand, because they have learned that it is in their own best interest not to admit it; the doctor is likely to act frustrated if they ask for something to be repeated.

Integrity rests on consistency between what the physician promises the patient and the outcome actually realized. Firm expectations are created in the patient's mind, which may turn out to have been unrealistic. The physician then makes the dangerous assumption that if something does go wrong, the patient can be expected to understand and to give the physician the opportunity to repair the damage. "After all, it's a rare complication and one that can be corrected with just one or two more procedures." The problem is this physician's tendency to oversimplify the issues. Establishing expectations that satisfy the patient's "wish" for a cure comes naturally. Yet if less than the promised outcome results, this physician cannot really apologize, as no room for errors or probabilities of less than fully satisfactory service were provided in the original description of services to be rendered. This physician has circumvented the communication required to share responsibility and to build trust, the kind of relationship that helps to create confidence and to prevent lawsuits.

Admitting failure goes against the grain and the 9,1-oriented physician may be tempted to hedge or blame some other member of the medical team for a failing that was actually predictable. This attitude of passing the buck rather than establishing realistic expectations in the first place is what makes this physician vulnerable.

Acquiring Knowledge. The 9,1-oriented physician sees knowledge as power and the key for exercising mastery and control. The rationale is never to get caught short by anyone. Medical school has inculcated the philosophy that ignorance cannot be excused and that total knowledge of a medical subject is an absolute necessity for the minimum standard of care.

This physician focuses on medical fact and ignores the human context of treatment. The answer to the question, "What are the unique circumstances in this patient's life that will affect my treatment?" is knowledge considered to be of little or no importance in the conduct of sound medical practice. Rather, a patient is a patient is a patient — existing for the sole purpose of being cured. Dr. Gray demonstrated the depth of his extensive medical knowledge to the residents and all of them were impressed with his dedication to the advancement of medical technology and technique, but it is unlikely he will ever learn that an intern reached out his hand for Mrs. Keating's hand, or the intensity of her response. Nor is it likely he will realize the extent to which he disregarded her humanity. Only that one intern learned a truly unforgettable lesson in the practice of sound medicine.

Assessing the patient's needs. Several factors do influence the approach that this physician takes to the treatment of a particular patient. One is the patient's ability to pay. If the patient is wealthy or has good insurance, then the physician can consider all possible procedures, as financial issues can be completely sidestepped.

Another factor related to satisfying the patient's medical needs concerns the availability of services. The service to be rendered is dependent to some degree on the medical facility, but the physician does not discuss these limitations in describing the services to be provided. The patient can either accept the physician's plan of treatment or go elsewhere. The truth is that the patient rarely is knowledgeable enough to know the limitations inherent in the services being offered. This physician's incentive is to stay busy, and therefore, the importance of a procedure or technique may be emphasized, even though this may refute the previously established expectations of the patient. The 9,1-oriented physician not only ignores the fact that the patient's need may be better met with a different technique that is not available in his or her hospital, but also sees no particular value in clarifying with the patient how facilities and equipment may limit the options available.

Decision Making. The 9,1-oriented physician believes that he or she alone has the required knowledge, experience, and authority to manage the medical situation at hand. Others are important only for their role in carrying out the decision.

Even though complications of treatment and therapy are a given in medicine, these physicians tend to blame circumstances or other personnel for any problem. The underlying 9,1 assumption remains, "I have the right answers, which encourages physicians to stand by decisions and defend them to all. Eventually facts may even be reinterpreted so that they support personal points of view, replacing conclusions consistent with objective data or the realities of the situation.

The 9,1-oriented physician, who needs to feel self-reliant and confident while making decisions, in time can be seen as rigid and heavy handed by patients and staff alike. Carried to an extreme, this physician can become the classic "bad doctor." Dogged persistence eliminates *needed* input by cutting out those who would offer contrary advice. Poor-quality care and genuine malpractice can result.

Level of responsibility. A level of responsibility is assumed by the physician and the patient in each physician-patient interaction. During typical interviews, the 9,1-oriented physician feels obligated to "take charge" and to assume all the responsibility for care. There is very little back-and-forth discussion of the type that leads to personal, logical decisions on the part of the patients about their care.

This physician does not comprehend that participation of the patients in the interview and treatment process can help focus the medical information and improve understanding and eagerness to cooperate. A nod or an acquiescent gesture is enough participation to satisfy this physician. Because patients are not invited to share a level of responsibility in their own care, they are more likely to feel that anything less than a perfect outcome is entirely the physician's fault.

Initiative. The 9,1-oriented manner of exercising initiative rests on three assumptions: 1) people want to be led, 2) telling others what to do is a powerful position, and 3) asking for suggestions demonstrates weakness or uncertainty. The unilateral exercise of initiative may go against the grain of some, but in the field of medicine it is seldom completely rejected. Many people are relieved by a physician's sense of control and willingness to guide them. Most will also respect the physician's ability to make things happen. "I drive myself and others; medicine is too important to do anything else" becomes a state of mind. The exercise of initiative itself is not resented, but rather the 9,1-oriented way of exercising that initiative: "I didn't ask for your advice; I asked for action." This approach reduces commitment and the ability of others to stay involved in the medical care being delivered.

Conflict Resolution. When conflict occurs, it is viewed as insubordination, something that must be suppressed, even put down by force if necessary. Suppression is a powerful means of extracting compliance, both from patients and the medical team. Counter-arguments are rejected as unacceptable. The physician pulls rank and announces the viewpoints that must prevail, with the expectation of obedience: "It is not important what you think. It is what you do that concerns me.

The difficulty of suppression as a method of resolving conflict is that it reveals a lack of confidence in the ability of others to act responsibly, and this can decrease their self-esteem and increase their resentment. In addition, more importantly for the physician, it eliminates the opportunity for individuals to make useful contributions as patients or members of the medical team.

Dealing with patient objections. Patients do not always agree with their physician's recommendations. Instead of using the patients' objections as warning signs of misunderstanding or of concerns that have not yet been explored, the physician triumphantly stamps "wrong" on the attitude of the patient and sets out to defeat the patient and to correct the error. This positive, overbearing attitude, reinforced by the extended technical vocabulary that the physician has at his or her disposal, can convince patients to forget or withhold objections. Another tactic is to ignore patients' objections altogether and to press on with the *important* medical information, often with a perturbed look, which says, "You're wasting my time."

There is no question that the 9,1-oriented physician attitude is a powerful one, and one that wins many patients to the particular procedure or service that the physician offers. However, the interaction does not build patient self-esteem or contribute to shared responsibility, and it may not create even a semblance of understanding. Too often the result is patient resentment and anger. A win-lose battle is on, and the blood that gets spilled is not likely to be the patient's.

Critique and Feedback. Feedback, a critical aspect of medical care, can be used by physicians to gauge their own effectiveness and to evaluate patient compliance. However, 9,1-oriented physicians do not take advantage of this valuable component of medical excellence. Confident of their own expertise, they do not feel the need for critique and feedback from patients or peers. The only sources of feedback for this physician are direct observation, inspection, and, on occasion, interrogation - a type of single-loop vigilance. Feedback has only one purpose: to be sure activities are proceeding according to his or her plan.

Informed consent. When patients question whether a treatment is in their own best interest, informed consent can become a potential mine field. In explaining the risks and benefits of a procedure with the contract before the patient, this physician attacks each objection with the presumption that, once every skirmish has been won, the patient has no alternative but to sign on the dotted line and to thus absolve the physician of responsibility for less than a perfect outcome. The patient has been led across a very shaky bridge to "informed consent."

The proceedings in a court of law can be used to illustrate the 9,1 approach to informed consent. The plaintiff's lawyer finds other 9,1-oriented physicians who sincerely believe, and are willing to say under oath, "There is only one treatment for this condition and all other techniques are malpractice." The defense attorney finds equally powerful physicians who support the procedure or service as actually delivered to the patient. The jury must listen to a whole series of 9,1-oriented physician approaches to the same medical condition and then decide if injury resulted, if negligence was demonstrated, and if financial reciprocation is justified as the "fair" solution. By removing responsibility from the patient, thinking of informed consent as a dictum for the only way to practice medicine, and living the 9,1 philosophy of "Not always right, but never in doubt," these physicians have distorted the concept of informed consent. Even if none of the physicians is wrong, the continued testimony of 9,1-oriented physicians against each other may push medical malpractice insurance rates to a point of limiting the delivery of medical care.

New and Established Patients

The 9,1-oriented physician tends to treat all patients alike, despite the fact that some are new and some are established. Building rapport is a necessity in both situations; however, these physicians feel that gaining rapport and trust lies in getting right down to brass tacks. After all, physicians represent expert opinion, and time is being wasted if idle chatter or personal involvement drifts into the patient-physician interaction. Trust evolves from credibility, and credibility is established through the display of vast knowledge.

When these physicians approach new patients, they demand attention from the opening line. Questions are posed that exclude the answer "no." Because these physicians do not like to be put off by idle questions, their goal is to present in precise detail the exact medical information necessary for each patient to agree with the treatment. At that point, these physicians consider optimal medical care to be underway.

With respect to established patients, these physicians assume that, because they have accepted the protection and benefits offered by their physician, they are literally the physician's property. The result is that 9,1-oriented physicians are even less involved with each individual's personal needs. The physician's attention is focused on those patients who require more technically sophisticated procedures or treatments. The rest of the patients are now given responsibility for their care, a role that has previously been denied them, and consequently follow-up and rehabilitation receive little attention until medical deterioration requires more complicated procedures to solve ongoing problems. These physicians feel the deterioration of the health of these patients results from poor compliance, yet the true cause lies in neglect of the needs of the individual.

Coping with the Busy Practice

Physicians who are 9,1 oriented are inner directed. They exercise control over personal actions, often using rigid self-prescriptions. This approach causes a blindness to unforeseen opportunities that surface during interactions with personnel and patients.

This physician tends to stay as busy as time and competition allow, creating a situation in which patients may wait for extended periods to take advantage of the most advanced medical techniques, surgical procedures, and treatments. You may have heard, "He has two appointment times, morning and afternoon, but it is worth the wait."

This physician tends to thrive on the rush of an overcrowded office with just one or two patients in excess of what would allow a work day free of fatigue. The justification is the self-held high value of the physician's skills. To have even a few empty chairs in the office or a few operative days unfilled is a waste of this physician's talents.

The 9,1-oriented physician is likely to think about his or her busy practice in the following ways:

Scheduling and Time Management. "I plan a fixed schedule of activities well in advance and I am damn good at not deviating from it. It has taken me years of experience to figure out how to do that. I use my valuable time with the patients to maximum advantage and do not tolerate any disturbances in the schedule."

The Hospital. "I make the hospital jump. I keep constant pressure on any area of weakness because the service I provide must always be the best."

Expenses. "I am ready to answer for every penny I spend in the delivery of medical care. These expenses are simply a means to an end. They are a requirement to be able to cure patients, and they are in line with the effort I put out to deliver medical care.

Continuing Education. "I read every article to support my point of view. I know the work of the experts by name. I push myself to be sure I'm always right."

Self-Evaluation. "I look at my records to be sure that I am busy; that means success. Beyond that, self-appraisal is not really necessary. It's diligent effort that makes a good physician. When I get ill, I take care of myself. After all, why not go to the best doctor?"

The 9,1 medical practice appears to be successful in that these physicians often remain very busy because of their take-charge attitude. They move fast, they exercise positive persuasion, and they brush aside objections and sweep patients into impetuous decisions to accept advice.

Recognizing 9,1 Behavior

The best way to identify the 9,1 orientation is to look at simple phrases in everyday language that describe this style:

Controls
Cuts people off
Drives hard
Exhibits impatience
Expects compliance
Finds fault
Gets into win-lose fights
Has all the answers
Interrogates
Is an exacting taskmaster
Is overpowering, stubborn, pushy, and quick to blame
Keeps others at a distance
Makes demands
Makes final decisions and tells people what to do
Sees things in black-and-white terms
Tells people what to do but not why
Is unable to listen

Patient Reactions Based On Grid Styles

What are the real consequences to the quality of care under this type of "successful" physician practice when viewed from the patient's perspective? Patient responses provide clues that are invaluable to the physician interested in developing a sounder medical practice.

The hard-driving approach of the 9,1-practicing physician generates two common responses: a disguised resentment for the physician because no opportunity is provided for patients to take personal responsibility, or active hostility and insult that lead patients to refuse care and to join the ranks of the many who confirm the faltering reputation of physicians as uncaring and arrogant. In addition to these two general reactions, more specific consequences of the 9,1 medical practice are dependent on each patient's Grid style.

9,1

Patients who are 9,1 oriented are exploitative and have as strong a drive to control as does the physician. They immediately assume that, like themselves, the physician will take advantage of the situation if given the opportunity. The 9,1-oriented physician, even though skilled at preventing questions, cannot control these patients. If the tone of the presentation of medical information is so persuasive as to raise the patient's suspicions, the patient may begin to ask loaded questions in order to test the physician. With many medical options available for the treatment of a particular disease, bolstered by both majority and minority opinions, the patient may hear an unexpected response, something that does not "square." Once the patient believes the physician is wrong or exaggerating, trust is destroyed, with little opportunity to regain it. A win-lose battle for control and domination is on. The physician tries to establish authority, and this patient remains unimpressed. Neither knuckles under.

Even if the physician creates some element of trust by arguments well defended or if the patient wins enough points to believe that a bargain is being offered, the tension in the interaction is inappropriate for a truly caring patient-physician relationship. More often than not, a stand-off results, and quality care is delayed or may not be delivered at all.

1,9

Patients who are 1,9 oriented are most likely to acquiesce to the 9,1-oriented physician. These patients are easy to satisfy and eager to please. Assuming that they will not understand much of the information that could be provided, the physician often goes straight to the benefits, knowing they are enough to satisfy these patients. He or she realizes these patients are unlikely to ask questions and is pleased that they create an opportunity to move through the busy office day more quickly.

The 1,9 attitude does not demand that specific needs actually be met, and the physician is unlikely to probe for realistic assessments of their situations. The difficulty comes in the fact that the patients' expectations reach an exaggeratedly high level regarding what the doctor and treatment can do for them. They admire the physician to such a great degree that they cannot imagine that he or she might ever fail them, and thus their reaction to failure is extreme disappointment. Their sense of betrayal leads, at the very least, to a quest for a new physician and, under extreme conditions, to lawsuits.

1,1

Patients who are 1,1 oriented are health burnouts. Their tendency is to withdraw from the medical situation, much as they have relinquished responsibility for their health care in the first place. They let the physician rattle off medical terminology, descriptions of surgical expertise, and cure rates, nonstop. Unencumbered, the 9,1-oriented physician continues until he or she is satisfied that an adequate level of information has been delivered, but rarely or never tests to see whether the patient understands.

These patients are likely to go along with whatever therapy the physician has described, particularly if the fit between the illness and the approach to cure is obvious. If for some reason they do not like the recommended treatment, they are likely to defer the decision on care.

If these patients demonstrate a lack of enthusiasm for nonstop advice, the physician may increase the pressure, closing in; and these patients may unexpectedly fight back, even with ferocity, angrily attacking the physician and stomping out of the office. Alternately, the patient may just take the easy way out, being lost to follow-up and continuing to deteriorate toward an emergency situation that requires no dialogue for care.

5,5

In order to feel secure, 5,5-oriented patients seek out physicians with a high degree of prestige: the "busy practice." They are most susceptible to the 9,1 approach if prominence is attached to the treatment and a number of illustrious people have been to the physician.

5,5-oriented patients approach medical interactions tentatively, uncertain of any kind of therapy except that acclaimed by their peers, highly touted medical journals, or preeminent medical experts. If these happen to be the 9,1-oriented physician's therapies of choice, these patients' needs may be met. However, an underlying fear that the services offered may not agree with their self-perception of need makes these patients sensitive to the physician who does not probe their desires in depth. Whether the physician eventually convinces the patients that the services are appropriate depends to a great degree on reputation.

Two difficulties with this type of physician-patient interaction can lead to poor quality care: One is that the patients' questions and interruptions are likely to be brushed aside. The second is that 5,5-oriented patients equally fear being taken advantage of and being criticized by the physician. The patients may feel that the physician is uncaring and is acting to embarrass them, and thus they may hedge on accepting the recommended treatment.

9,9

Patients who are 9,9 oriented approach the physician-patient interaction with an interest in sound consultation. The 9,1-oriented physician, concentrating on medical knowledge, stimulates these patients' interests. They can be expected to question the physician at points where information does not agree with their factual knowledge or assessment of the situation. If the 9,1-oriented physician tries to diminish the importance of these checkpoints or to brush objections aside, the patients will persist until questions are satisfactorily answered. Although, when challenged, the physician may attempt to convert the interview into a win-lose argument, these patients are likely to maintain composure and to continue probing for information to help them in making informed decisions about their own care. If the physician cannot explain the medical service to the satisfaction of these patients, they are likely to seek information elsewhere, going from one physician to another until an effective bridge of communication can be constructed.

Even though 9,9-oriented patients are the most adequately prepared to genuinely participate in health care delivery, the likelihood of their receiving optimal care from the 9,1-oriented physician is unpredictable. If the physician's service meets the patients' self-formulated requirements, then acceptable care results. If not, the physician probably lacks the flexibility required to view the patients' needs and provide good medical care. The physician's opportunity to care for these patients is lost, but with persistence and time, these patients enter the health care delivery system successfully, even if some disillusionment about physicians is picked up along the way.

Summary

The 9,1-oriented physician's attitude can be summed up as hard working, apparently self-assured, high technology, and procedure oriented. This physician is all work, no play, no interruptions, no irrelevancies. He or she is generally quite powerful, both in presence and in position. Yet this practice style undercuts the role of the individual in critical life episodes. What are lost are the physician's role of support and caring, the richness of warm human understanding, and the ability to sense how the patient is feeling — the true art of medicine.

The overall consequences of the 9,1 orientation in the delivery of medical care are a lack of trust and creation of expectations greater than can be guaranteed by the sophistication of medicine. The approach of this physician provides the grist for the media industry to describe the physician as, at times, blatantly exploitative of the patient. A sense of apparent helpfulness is seen as a cover-up for ever greater numbers of medical treatments, sophisticated surgical procedures, and skyrocketing medical costs. The 9,1 set of assumptions erodes trust because the entire approach has lost the human touch. Without earned trust, the patient's positive attitude toward medical care can be easily converted into resentment and long-lasting antagonism toward physicians in general.

When inadequate skills make understanding patients' personal needs difficult and sometimes impossible, the physician may find success shallow, and achievement may begin to lose its reward. For this physician, life affords few pleasures. There is only work and, with persistence, retirement never comes.

Chapter Five

1,9 MEDICAL CARE: BUILDING THE PRACTICE WITH A SMILE

"Hi, Roy. It's good to see you. I was wondering about you and Jean just the other day. How is the family?"

Roy grasped his stomach, leaned forward, and smiled in his usual manner, for just a moment forgetting the pain that had brought him into the doctor's office.

"How are you doing, Roy? I hear you're having a little belly pain." Dr. Walters placed his hand on Roy's back with a genuine look of concern.

"Well, Stu, I've had this pain ever since I ate two pork chops last night. I wasn't able to sleep all night, and I've never felt anything like it in all my 68 years."

Dr. Walters leaned back with a reassuring look, pleased to be on a first name basis, "Well, Roy, these things aren't usually a problem. We just need to take a look and make sure everything is OK." Again, he reached out and patted Roy on the back as he moved to the door of the exam room. 'Just go ahead and change there, Roy, and I'll be back in to do your exam." Roy kind of leaned over and began to undress as Dr. Walters left the room.

Being careful not to keep the patient waiting, Dr. Walters returned to the examination room, which was well decorated, exuding a wand and comfortable atmosphere. Roy was lying on his back in a cloth gown as Dr. Walters approached his right side and placed his hand over the area of the liver. "Is this where it hurts, Roy?"

"Yeah, that's it, Doc."

"Well, sounds like you've got a gallbladder problem to me. Don't worry.

These things happen all the time and we may not have to do anything but limit the amount of fat in your diet. If it really gets bad, then we will just take it out."

Roy's faint smile faded to a grimace at the thought of surgery. Dr. Walters stopped, noting the change in expression. "Don't worry, Roy, we probably won't have to operate." Dr. Walters shook Roy's hand and concluded, "Stop in my office so I can give you a bland diet and some Tylenol."

* * * * *

Six months later Roy returned to Dr. Walter's office, in pain once more. "That pain is back, Stu. I did everything you said Dr. Walters, almost overly eager, interrupted, "Oh, no, I'm really sorry to hear that. Tell me exactly what happened."

"Well, it's probably my own fault. I did have just one pork chop, with a little gravy, but basically I've done everything you said. Why isn't the diet working?"

"Roy, it's not your fault. Everybody cheats on a diet, but that's when the old gallbladder acts up. You've got a fever this time so we need to do some tests."

Dr. Walters poked his head out the door to his nurse, "Pam, call over to X-ray and set up an upper GI and ultrasound of the gallbladder." He turned back to Roy, "You could just have an ulcer, so I'm going to start you on Tagamet and give you some ampicillin for the fever. Why don't you get dressed, and I will check with Pam to be sure they can get you in today. Just stop in my office so we can talk about the test before you go over. I want to explain the procedures so they will be a little easier on you.

Feeling reassured by two new medications and Dr. Walters' sensitivity, Roy left for the hospital. When he returned a few days later to discuss the results of the tests, Dr. Walters smiled, "Gee, Roy, you look great."

"Well I don't feel great."

"What's wrong? What happened?" Sensing that Roy was not only ill but angry, Dr. Walters moved closer and extended his hand.

As Roy automatically took Dr. Walters' hand, he felt the genuine warmth of their long relationship. He sighed deeply as his anger subsided and said, "When I got to X-ray they told me you should have ordered a different test, so I had to take these pills and go back the next day. As if that wasn't enough! Nothing showed up so I had to do the whole thing again. What's going on?"

Dr. Walters, trying to hide his discomfort, evaded his question. "Let me go check; something's not right here." He returned with the results of the double-dose oral cholecystogram and explained. "These tests are always run when the other tests are normal, so everything was done just like it should have been."

Roy remained expressionless.

"The important thing is that we are going to get you back to your family and work."

Roy nodded and said, "Boy, I hope so. I still feel miserable."

"Well, Roy, you've definitely got gallstones and it looks like they're infected. We probably better get those things out of there."

"Please, Stu, I really don't want to have surgery and I can't afford it. I'd

rather just wait and see if we can't tough this thing out. Can't you give me some more antibiotics?"

Dr. Walters leaned back and reassessed the situation. "Well, Roy, it's going to be risky to wait this out, but if you feel like surgery is not for you, you're the boss and we'll try a conservative approach."

Roy smiled, "Yeah, I think I'll be all right. Everybody in my family has had gallstones, and they've all had them removed. My brother almost died from complications when they did surgery. I'd just like to avoid that if I can."

Dr. Walters patted Roy on the back, shook his hand firmly, and commiserated, "I can understand that. We'll do everything we can to be sure that you don't have the same problems that your brother did. You know, Roy, it amazes me how good you look, even when you're sick." Roy smiled. "Say hello to Jean for me, and tell that grandson of yours, Bob, that I'm looking forward to seeing him play in the football game this Saturday."

Roy looked up and smiled with the recognition that Dr. Walters really did remember his entire family. He felt comforted, knowing that he was in good hands. Yet he walked out the door still guarding his right side, inexplicably afraid that something was wrong. As the pain resolved over the next few weeks and he felt better, Roy's fear diminished. Only his sudden death, not too long after, revealed that a time bomb, still ticking inside him, should have been removed.

General Characteristics of the 1,9-Orientation to Medicine

The 1,9 orientation is shown in the upper left-hand corner of the Grid, where technical excellence is abandoned for the sake of a legitimately high concern for people. These physicians, if challenged, seriously question whether the cure is worth the social stress on the patient. Their general assumption is that technical expertise often conflicts with the needs and desires of real people. The choice of therapy may be based on the desire to satisfy personal needs, even if the accepted standard of care has to be bent a little in the process.

Physicians who are 1,9 oriented are often hard working, carrying a large patient load and willing to expend a great deal of effort to meet the emotional needs of the patient, as well as remember details of his or her family, job, likes, and dislikes. They are willing to talk at great length if that will help a scared patient population confront the critical life-and-death diagnoses that are a part of everyday medical practice.

Motivation

The 1,9-motivated physician gains no real enjoyment from the procedure well done or the medical achievement of good therapy, but is driven by the need to generate and maintain harmony. This physician feels secure only when the physician-patient relationship is "going well." The physician is sensitive to what the patient thinks and can be described as tender hearted, helpful, kind, and sympathetic. When the patient shows appreciation, a general feeling of high satisfaction and success pervades the medical practice. To achieve this goal, this physician is motivated to create an atmosphere of warmth and caring.

The negative side of the 1,9-oriented physician's motivation is a fear of disapproval or rejection. A typical reaction to this fear is avoiding what the patient does not like, the most classic examples being pelvic and rectal examinations. The patient is unlikely to request an unpleasant procedure or physical evaluation, and if a tumor or major medical problem is missed, the patient is rarely knowledgeable enough to know that the reason may be neglect of a routine part of the physical evaluation.

When a 1,9 orientation spreads throughout a hospital or a medical care team, the atmosphere resembles a country club, where people are agreeable and express high levels of satisfaction, but the problem is that medical techniques and routines are manipulated to keep everyone happy. A 1,9 orientation, unresolved, results in poor-quality medical care and may be the source of legitimate medical malpractice.

The 1,9-Oriented Physician-Patient Relationship

Providing Patient Care

The one consistent component of patient care for the 1,9-oriented physician is the sincere desire to affirm each patient's value as a person. This overly solicitous attitude to the patient results in wandering from the point and interviews stretching out to an indeterminable length. Rather than concentrating on accurate diagnosis, this physician directs his concern elsewhere, and the decisiveness typical of medical excellence is lost.

Communication. With a 1,9 style of communication, the physician views nothing as black and white, and there is always room for discussion. The physician gauges the appropriate response to questions by whether hostility or friendliness is perceived as the underlying motivation. interruptions are treated with the utmost interest and respect. However, the patient may perceive this attitude as too soft, lacking the strength of convictions expected from a physician. Carried to an extreme, the lengthy conversation may be viewed as irrelevant. The patient may have come to the physician seeking food for thought but leaves feeling only tranquilized.

Establishing patient expectations. The 1,9-oriented physician sees medical therapy as less precise than do most physicians and, thus, avoids establishing anything beyond minimum expectations in the mind of the patient. If direct questions imply a higher expectation than can be "guaranteed," this physician will not disappoint the patient but will carefully sidestep by saying, "We will do our best. Medicine isn't a perfect science. We haven't learned it all, but you are in a much better place than you would have been 50 years ago. Now we have the tests, the antibiotics, and the surgical skills to give you the very best chance at getting through this difficulty. But medicine holds no guarantees." And at that point, with a reassuring smile and physical contact through either a handshake or a pat on the back, the patient has truly been given a reasonable expectation of medicine's limitations. This may be one of the high points of this style.

One difficulty with establishing patient expectations is that admitting failure may come too easily to this physician. If the outcome is not what was discussed in the preliminary patient-physician encounter, this well-meaning physician is tempted to offer a refund or a price reduction. This is unwarranted, in that the medical care was delivered, regardless of the outcome. However, the expectation that builds in the patient is that the physician must be offering a refund because an error was committed.

Acquiring Knowledge. To the 1,9-oriented physician, knowledge means knowing the patient. Oftentimes a physician will gather information about the patient prior to their first meeting. This can be done by the nursing staff, who will put special notes in the patient's chart, such as who referred the patient, what the family situation is, and what the particular social concerns are, in addition to the reason for the medical visit. This concern for the human side of the patient is commendable, yet when the physician becomes preoccupied with these details, he or she is less likely to develop a deep knowledge or understanding of the medical issues at hand.

Attention to the practice style of other physicians is minimal. When patients describe treatments they have heard about elsewhere, the physician is uninterested and this blind spot becomes obvious. The patient may lose faith in the physician, despite the personal attention.

The physician who persists in a 1,9 orientation to medical practice eventually becomes technically uninformed. Dr. Walters exemplifies the physician who can look good even though medical practice is suffering. He has learned what he can "get away with" to please the patient without causing a medical disaster that will be linked directly to therapy he has advised. In the issue of a cholecystitis with documented gallstones, conservative therapy, quieting the inflammation prior to a surgical approach, is acceptable. However, another option is to operate in the face of the low-grade inflammation because of the excellent antibiotic coverage available and because of the increased risk of subsequent attacks in someone over 65. Dr. Walters falls somewhere in between. He treated the patient conservatively, accepting the patient's fear of surgery as reasonable, vowing to do everything he could to prevent the disaster that befell Roy's brother. Yet when Roy's death occurred, one could legitimately track its cause back to the physician who did not appropriately encourage the patient to eliminate the risk of complications by indicated surgery.

The 1,9-oriented physician commonly gets much positive feedback from patients, who, indeed, understand and appreciate personal attention more than medical expertise. The bottom line is that the physician acquires very little of the knowledge needed as a basis for making sound shared decisions about medical care.

Assessing the patient's needs. Evaluation of the patient need is dependent on whether the patient demonstrates approval of the information-gathering process. The attitude of a patient who is ill at ease or impatient automatically cuts the interview short. Inquiry tends to be shallow when it relates to assessing medical needs and to be deep in terms of human needs.

Monetary factors also have a great impact on the information-gathering process. If certain lab tests or therapies are out of the economic range of the patient because he or she is "self-pay" or uninsured, the physician, realizing the financial and therefore emotional burden that would be imposed on the patient, is not likely to suggest them. Financial considerations may also tempt a generalist to provide care that would be more appropriately delivered by a specialist, never realizing that the expertise of the specialist may be therapeutic, or at times even lifesaving for the patient, despite its higher cost. Concern for the human side of the patient may override an accurate analysis of the patient's total needs.

Defining the patient's medical needs may also be affected if the physician lacks updated knowledge on what services are available in the community or even at the physician's hospital. The physician's intention is to stay busy on the basis of popularity. As the years pass, the physician develops the fine art of realizing what needs can be met within his or her fund of knowledge. No effort is made to compare alternative therapies provided by other institutions or other specialties.

Decision Making. The 1,9-oriented physician may recognize that he or she does not have the knowledge and experience to manage the medical side of a certain situation alone. He or she is likely then to ask a specialist for a "curbside consultation" and to use the information gathered in making a medical decision, even if the presentation to the specialist does not exactly reflect the patient situation. This sense of having obtained a consultation prior to decision making encourages the physician to keep the patient, reassures the family, and may allow the situation to evolve into a major emergency.

Another solution to difficult or unpopular decisions is to postpone them, in areas that cause anxiety for the physician due to a deficient medical background, the physician may not respond to the patient's needs because subconsciously he or she would prefer to be involved in a more pleasant discussion with another patient who has a simpler problem. The hope is that, by delay, the medical situation will become clearer or a favorable situation will replace the poor progress that is at hand. A common example is when antibiotics are used in view of a clinically unresponsive infection. The physician simply continues them, hoping that, finally, after even four or five days of spiking temperatures, spiraling white counts, and deterioration of vital signs, the clinical picture will somehow improve. The family and patient are likely to share the physician's genuine concern and worry about the individual who has become ill, yet these physicians, because of the leadership style that emerges when faced with a decision, commonly wait for a crisis in hopes of a clearer perception of the best response. if we were to analyze the actual situation, the decision in question probably never did get made; rather, the patient moved beyond it to a new series of diagnoses and complications.

Level of responsibility. Shared responsibility is the key phrase for the 1,9-oriented physician. The sense of togetherness established from the start replaces the take-charge attitude of many physicians. The extended discussions that ensue should lead to personal, logical decisions; however, the physician delivers only partial information, as the fund of knowledge is inadequate to do otherwise. The friendly atmosphere created is unsuitable for life-and-death decisions and the compelling business at hand. instead, it resembles a coffee break visit, which is fine as long as the patient was not actually ill in the first place. Although the physician feels good, the patient is not constructively aided so as to become more capable of self-care.

Initiative. The assumptions that direct initiative from the 1,9 orientation are 1) the patient is always right, 2) medical technology is not what it is cracked up to be and is expensive, and 3) meeting the patient's emotional need in a life crisis is more important than proceeding logically with the medical therapy. This physician is not a leader. However, lack of initiative in carrying out medical plans is balanced by high initiative in gaining bonds of friendship, further contacts, and an ever greater patient population.

Patients seldom question the physician's exercise of initiative when all activity is directed toward making them feel better. However, in an era of peer review and continuing medical education as a requirement for malpractice insurance, inconsistent medical technique, outmoded therapy, or inappropriate medical treatment at the request of a patient is easily discovered. The quality of medical care becomes unreliable and at times even dangerous, eliminating the ability of technically well-trained medical personnel to support the physician locked into this type of practice.

Conflict Resolution. The 1,9-oriented physician has a critical need to sidestep real conflict. Conversations are actually steered away from topics that might provoke controversy or ill feelings. If questions do arise, they are quickly smoothed over or bypassed: "That's an important question, and I'm going to get to that, but I want to deal with how you're feeling. I can tell you're concerned." The physician, who often has a good sense of humor, may make light of the issue, telling a joke, easing tensions, patting the patient on the back, and underplaying what the patient knows to be a serious problem. It is almost impossible to engage in an argument with a 1,9-oriented physician. Patients may remain silent finally, rather than cause this physician, whom they truly do like, any embarrassment. The final result is the same — less than optimal quality medical care.

Dealing with patient objections. If the patient has objections or misunderstandings, the physician is likely to delve into the personal reasons behind the misinterpretation, genuinely perceiving fear or the discomfort of an aggravating disease, yet avoiding what the patient really came for: highly competent medical advice. Because the physician creates an environment steeped with warmth and affection, patients are often mollified. Yet it is the physician's direct response to objections, interruptions, complaints, and questions about medical techniques that aids the patient in establishing a firm conviction about a particular treatment.

If the problem ultimately must be dealt with, despite the anticipated resentment, the physician reveals a little at a time to achieve a sugar-coated effect. This physician fears that explaining the blunt truth all at once could produce an explosion and a loss of the bond that has been nurtured over the entire course of the patient-physician relationship.

This physician also apologizes when an outcome is less than optimal. To relieve feelings of rejection, the physician may suggest additional minor treatments or follow-ups, emphasizing the time commitment he or she is willing to make to ensure that this patient has a full recovery despite the "minor complication" that has occurred.

Critique and Feedback. Closely related to objections is critique and feedback, which the 1,9-oriented physician is excellent at obtaining and dealing with, often at length. Through keen skills of emotional observation, the 1,9-oriented physician monitors patient satisfaction, rather than using critique and feedback to check the physician's own effectiveness or patient compliance. The physician has a long history of positive feedback and is relatively assured that "good vibes" will come from questions like, "How do you feel compared to a few months ago when you didn't know whether your condition might be fatal?" or "Isn't it amazing that only a hundred years ago you might even have died from this disease. Doesn't it make you feel lucky?" The key to this physician's feedback scheme is that it is directed toward gaining the acceptance and reinforcing the bonds that are so important to maintain a 1,9 orientation. Criticisms are sidestepped or written off as misunderstandings, and the real benefits of self-analysis are lost.

Informed consent. The shared responsibility that evolves from the 1,9-oriented physician style should lend itself to ideal informed consent. One factor prevents this from being true, however: the content of information delivered may not be up to date or comprehensive, but rather reflects what that physician feels will meet the emotional needs of the patient. In explaining the risks and benefits of surgery or some other medical therapy, the 1,9-oriented physician downplays the real medical risks so as to avoid scaring the patient and provides information that is heavily influenced by the emotional tone of the patient during the interview.

An important point to remember about this physician is the patient's genuine belief that the physician will fulfill the expectations that have been established. Therefore, the physician feels no need to worry the patient by describing possible complications and may even make the critical mistake of saying, "Yes, I am sure this treatment will meet all of your requirements." Actual misrepresentation may be the result of this attitude, but it is by no means a conscious deception on the part of the physician.

The principles of informed consent have been met to the best of the physician's ability and have been understood to the best of the patient's ability. The difficulty arises in the complicated case where less than a perfect outcome results. At that point, an in-depth quality assurance investigation of the medical-technical care will follow. When it becomes clear that alternative medical therapies were not mentioned or that a better medical treatment may have been available, the conclusion is that informed consent for that particular procedure or therapy was not part of the physician-patient dialogue.

New and Established Patients

To get and keep patients, a physician must establish good rapport as well as a good reputation in the community. The 1,9-oriented physician becomes acquainted with the patient in a comfortable atmosphere and takes the time to establish a secure feeling of acceptance prior to delving into the patient's problem. The 1,9-oriented assumption is that patients go to the physician who can best take care of their problems and that patients really are not very interested in the medical-technical aspects of health care delivery. At the conclusion of each interview, the physician is likely to thank the patient for selecting him or her as a health care provider, reassuring the patient that everything within the physician's power will be done to take care of this patient for as long as the patient lives and the physician remains in practice.

The new patient is unlikely to perceive that the physician is short on medical knowledge. The established patient, however, has had a longer exposure to the physician, and hiding an inadequate technical background becomes a challenge. The solution for the 1,9-oriented physician is to establish minimum expectations, to sidestep, and to recount the limitations of medicine in general. Having never established high technical expectations, this physician rarely has to deal with a patient who feels expectations have been violated. Any mistake brings profuse apologies regarding the human aspect of the practice of medicine and the physician's personal sorrow over the situation. This quality of empathy oftentimes is valued more highly than the competence of the technical expert who arrogantly keeps patients at a distance and accepts no guilt.

Coping with the Busy Practice

The 1,9-oriented physician spends a lot of time with both established and new patients, enjoying the relationships that have been formed with them. This physician believes that social contacts are necessary for success in practice, especially in these days of high competition, and these contacts are assiduously cultivated both in and out of the office. Names are memorized and used frequently to demonstrate how important each patient is to the physician. As word of this attentiveness spreads, business grows. The excessive time expended in this approach is rationalized by the results it brings. The 1,9-oriented physician is less keen about patients who are abrupt, abrasive, or demanding, and therefore spends less time with those individuals. Slowly culling them out of the practice, this physician allows them to become lost to follow- up in hopes that they will not return when their expectations are unfulfilled.

Because the 1,9-oriented physician does not wish to risk the patient's displeasure by saying "no," he or she makes multiple commitments until the busy state of the practice precludes these commitments being fulfilled. Although the physician's promises are sincere, "I'll do everything I can to meet your wishes," "Of course, I'll take calls; just phone my home and I'll come in and take care of you," they cannot always be met. Only later, when unfulfilled expectations can be connected to a less-than-perfect medical outcome, is the extent of the patient's disappointment realized. If the physician is aware of being overextended, he or she begins to rationalize: "Well, I had an emergency, and I just couldn't get over to see you." "We did everything that was possible, but sometimes even everything isn't enough." "I feel bad about having disappointed you, but that's the limitation of the system. I did everything I could." "What can I do for you now? I've always tried to do the best I could by you. I think you know that." Patients may be kept waiting for hours, but they are appeased because they believe in the sincerity of their physician and they desperately want someone to care about the feeling of ill health that has brought them to the medical system.

The following depicts ways the 1,9-oriented physician copes with a busy practice:

Scheduling and Time Management. "I am at my patients' disposal. My work schedule has flexibility so I can help them when they need me. Sometimes this keeps me from being available to my family, but I'm doing everything I can."

The Hospital. "Medical teamwork is everything. We have to work together, we have to care about each other and be friends to provide the top-notch medical care we're all capable of. I don't hesitate to ask for help. Even the nurses and the patients have worthwhile opinions about how care should be delivered."

Expenses. "We need to do everything we can to keep the patient's expenses down. The physician who orders laboratory tests without first considering whether the patient can afford them should reconsider the service being provided in this highly technical era. As for my expenses, no expense is too large to create a pleasant and reassuring atmosphere for the patient."

Continuing Education. "I get my education on the job. My years of experience have taught me more than those erudite rat studies that everybody keeps quoting. I do feel that we are obligated to use patient education brochures and all of the material that's available to help the patient stay involved in the care we provide."

Self-Evaluation. "My evaluation comes from the patients. Their love and dedication are constant reminders to me of the good medical care I have provided over the years. I am in tune with patient reactions, and I do whatever is needed to increase their acceptance of me. Caring leads to good medical care."

Recognizing 1,9 Behavior

Simple phrases characterize this set of assumptions and physician style. The following list will help you recognize the 1,9 orientation:

Agreeable
Appreciative
Considerate

Eager for harmony
Easily hurt
Excessively complimentary
Nice
Overly eager
Overly trusting
Sensitive
Supportive and comforting
Uncomfortable with disagreement
Uncontroversial
Unlikely to probe
Willing to hear what others think before speaking
Willing to yield to gain approval

Patient Reactions Based On Grid Styles

The 1,9-oriented physician's degree of success is linked to the patient and the style that the patient uses in seeking out medical care.

9,1

A 9,1-oriented patient's attitude of strength, domination, and even suspicion conveys hostility and rejection to the 1,9-oriented physician. The physician may initially try to respond with friendliness, jokes, and the usual warmth that wins so many patients. However, when these techniques are rejected, the physician beats a hasty withdrawal. The encounter may be extremely brief, with the physician simply stating, "I don't think I'll be able to meet your needs," closing the patient chart, and leaving the room.

If the physician is able to create trust through sincere warmth and concern, the trade-off will be giving the 9,1-oriented patient total authority over medical decision making. This combination can be mutually satisfying as long as all goes well. However, this patient's solution to poor-quality care or to failed expectations is likely to be confrontation and, in extreme cases, a lawsuit.

1,9

The 1,9-oriented physician approach is understandably most successful with a 1,9-oriented patient in that the need of each individual to be liked is certain to be satisfied. Mutual admiration and friendliness prevail, as the encounter becomes essentially a social visit. The difficulty is that such a relationship may never address the issue at hand. The patient may leave the doctor's office never having asked the critical questions that took him or her there in the first place.

If medical advice is rendered, it will almost surely be accepted for the sake of the relationship, even if it is of poor quality and unsound when tested against needs or expectations.

1,1

The 1,1-oriented patient is burned out and responds to the 1,9 presentation with noncommittal answers and a lack of interest. The physician is disturbed by the unresponsive patient's impact on the normally pleasant physician-patient relationship. One reaction may be to search for a mutual social interest; but if the social backgrounds are widely separated, as when the patient is from a low socioeconomic group, the patient is more likely to be abandoned. Alternatives are offered, as the physician genuinely tries to find someone who can take care of this difficult patient.

5,5

The 5,5-oriented patient is quite happy as long as all of his or her friends have been satisfied with the same treatment. Because the 1,9-oriented physician inspires little confidence in this patient, the physician may become discouraged and ill at ease. The physician's memory of well-known patients who were satisfied may be used to bolster the relationship. if the physician emphasizes caring rather than the treatment that is in vogue, with a poor outcome the patient may lose confidence in the physician.

9,9

The 9,9-oriented patient is likely to feel frustrated with the irrelevancy and soft content of what the 1,9-oriented physician has to say. The slow progress and lack of solid medical facts that characterize the 1,9 medical style simply do not meet the solution-seeking requirements of this patient. The 9,9 orientation stands the best chance of moving this physician toward a style more compatible with that of medical excellence. If this effort fails, the physician will find the interaction uncomfortable, but is unlikely to understand why the 9,9-oriented patient does not reciprocate with friendliness and congeniality. If the patient is thorough in the process of information gathering, the physician's lack of medical skill will be obvious, and the patient will seek another physician who ensures the opportunity to participate in excellent medical care.

Summary

Physicians who are 1,9 oriented are easy to characterize.In everything they do, their desire is to help and support others. They work toward harmony, look for facts and beliefs that suggest all is well, and at the same time trust that all will go well. They avoid generating conflict by searching for decisions that will maintain good relations and by encouraging others to make decisions for themselves. Positive in their orientation, they find criticism of others as difficult as being wrong themselves. They understand how the patient is feeling but have lost the power and presence of truly high-quality technical decision making.

Improving technical skills requires time, a break from the routine that has created this physician style, and a dedication to the medical excellence that is within reach of this physician group. The needed continuing medical education is more than just a challenge for this physician. The inevitable result of this practice style without this shift in attitude will be years of dedicated practice that fall short of the good reputation to which these physicians aspire. As medical expertise and new information spiral past them, they will become the "old timers" everybody looks out for. Ultimately they will feel that the profession of medicine, as well as many of their faithful trusted patients, has abandoned them.

Chapter Six

9+9 MEDICAL CARE: FATHER KNOWS BEST

Dr. Marcia Welby walked into the nurses' station, having the air of someone regal in her long white coat and silver hair. Over the years, she had distinguished herself as a learned, mature leader in the medical community. She had long since gotten over the jokes about her name being so much like that of the silver-haired mentor whom she had emulated in her early career. She had always found the joking somewhat complimentary. Although some might have dismissed Dr. Welby as the kind of unrealistic portrayal one expected from television, he had some pretty darn good qualities.

"Hi, Jill. How's it going, Donna?" Reaching for the nursing log, she smiled and gave a nod of recognition to each nurse.

The jokes that the Welby name had triggered in Marcia's early career like, "Who does she think she is, Dr. Welby?" or "That may work on television, but not here," had been replaced by comments like, "This is the real Dr. Welby. Marcus couldn't hold a candle to her."

Marcia looked up from the nursing log and called Jill back to the nurses station. "Now, Jill, you know better than this. Look at these vital signs. They've been put in the wrong column, and it looks like you've left off all of the temperature charting. And what about the I and O that I ordered?"

Jill looked up, struggling to contain a rebuttal. She glanced around the nurses' station and noted the disapproval registered by her peers, who were clearly siding with Marcia. They had all learned that Marcia rewarded loyalty, so it was the wise thing to do. And beyond that, they knew she meant well, even when they found her style offensive.

"Now I know you didn't do this on purpose, Jill, and I'm sure you'll do better in the future," Dr. Welby went on. She patted Jill on the shoulder as she turned to walk away, and Jill mimicked a cowering puppy as a protest to Marcia's patronizing approach.

People who didn't measure up to her expectations were a trial for Dr. Welby. The previous day she had been called to the emergency room, where she had met a GI bleeder. The call schedule required her to admit the patient under her name and to take the initial steps to stabilize him prior to the surgeon's decision about whether this chronic alcoholic, who had already had several hospitalizations, should have a portal-caval shunt. Dr. Welby felt that medical management of patients like this should be conservative, considering the fact that the patient was never going to be responsible enough to take care of himself and that extensive and expensive treatment was therefore just a waste. The patient's name was Tom something. Dr. Welby was not too good on last names, but seemed to know everybody's first name and nickname in most cases. As she moved into Tom's room, it was clear that he was angry.

"Well, Tom, what have you done now? Here you are back in the hospital. What are we going to do with you?"

Tom just glared at Dr. Welby. "Well, for one thing, you can get this damn tube out of my nose.

"Now, now, now. You know this is for your own good, Tom. We're just trying to save you from yourself."

Tom sat straight up and said, "If you don't pull this tube out, I'm going to take it out myself. I'm getting out of this place. You people don't have any idea how to treat me anyway.

"Well, Tom, you can do whatever you want. I mean, everybody here has bent over backwards for you. We take you off the street, bring you in here through the emergency room, give you blood, and for what? So that you can go back out on the streets, get drunk, and be back here all over again."

At that point Tom disconnected the suction tube from the wall and started to put on his pants.

"Now, now, Tom, calm down, calm down. I'll get the nurses. We need you back in bed." Dr. Welby turned and rushed out of the room, and called, "Jill, Donna, please get in there and take care of Tom what's-his-name. I think he's going to leave AMA." Dr. Welby turned to the remaining nurse; she was dutifully standing her post at the nurses' station, covering the phone and watching the lights on the automated systems that would let her know if any patients were in trouble. Dr. Welby fully expected Jill and Donna to go into the room and sort things out. They had played this role for her before, and she had come to depend on it.

Karin, who was manning the nurses' station, smiled and said, "He's kind of a tough one, isn't he?"

Dr. Welby looked up, stuck out her chest, and threw her head back. "Well, there was a day when patients listened to you. I got up in the middle of the night to help this guy; I'm on a call schedule to take care of people like this, and I don't mind as long as they're grateful. We save their lives over and over again, and what do we get? Nothing in return." She shook her head and began walking down the hallway.

She sighed as she realized that that encounter would make her late to her office. She had a handful of informed consent forms that she was taking to the office so that she could get them signed while the patients were getting their *routine exams. Her thought was to have them simply sign the forms for whatever care she decided was best for the patients. That made a lot of sense to Dr. Welby, as her popularity meant that her office was always slightly overcrowded. Informed consent was really just a formality; after all, she was the last word in the care for her patients. Her decision would stand, as the very nature of her relationship with her patients implied informed consent. So this step would meet the hospital requirements and smooth things out on rounds.*

She vowed that she would never take care of this Tom character again. He had insulted her and had been incapable of the slightest respect. As she passed the emergency room on her way out of the hospital, she reflexively turned and went directly into the supervisor's office, where she expressed her frustration at trying to care for patients like Tom — Tom Parker, that was his name — who didn't want to be helped.

The supervisor started to comment several times and realized that it wasn't really worth it. Preachers weren't partial to interruptions in the middle of their sermons. The appropriate role for the supervisor was to sit back and nod knowingly, letting the great Dr. Welby ventilate.

"I know it's not your fault, Bill. I mean, rules are rules, and we do have to take call. I just want it posted somewhere that I don't feel I'm capable of meeting his needs. I think he's just waiting for somebody to screw up so that he can sue all of us."

Bill began to speak and Marcia quickly interrupted.

"And if he's going to sue anybody, it's going to be me. He's up there right now throwing one of his tantrums, threatening to pull the nasal-gastric tube out and storm back to the streets, no doubt for a quick bottle of Thunderbird."

Bill began to nod. "Yes, yes. Okay, Marcia, I understand."

Marcia wheeled around and, with her coat flying behind her, proceeded out of the hospital.

Something had happened. The system just wasn't supporting her like it used to. People questioned her now, when before they simply stood at attention and said, "Yes, ma'am," or in some cases, "Yes, sir." Somehow people no longer had the proper respect for the field of medicine, even for those individuals who were clearly above average, like herself. She had been in practice for 25 years and this year, for the first time, had gotten sued — and the patient was one she liked and who she thought liked her. That had really hurt her feelings. In fact, the lawsuit had led her to consider whether this should be her last year in practice. But then what would she do? Medicine was her life. Taking care of her "children," as she called them, was what she lived for. Maybe the system would change, maybe things would get better. At least there were still those patients who understood and valued the care she provided. They would always be grateful for the time she took to reach out and touch them and help them through the medical crises that brought so much suffering to so many. That's what made her life worth living and, for them, she would stay in practice.

General Characteristics of the
9+9-Orientation to Medicine

One leadership style, paternalism or the coaching model, is a major force in medicine. The assumption is that the coach knows what's best for the team and therefore takes the responsibility of coordinating all of their activities. We call this style 9+9, as it is the style that draws a connection between 1,9 and 9,1. The 9+9 medical style could be shown graphically on the Grid by an arc connecting the 1,9 and 9,1 corners. This approach is an either/or combination of a high concern for the cure alternated with a high concern for people. It does not imply an integration of the two concerns as in a 9,9 orientation, but rather an additive combination of the two. The basic assumption of the physician toward a patient is, "I am responsible for you and want to help you (much as if the other person were a son or daughter). In return, I expect your loyalty as a matter of course."

Even though the style is referred to as paternalism, it is in no way limited by gender. Women like Marcia Welby who have the 9+9 style tend to exhibit the characteristics of a father figure, complete with authority and all-knowing control, rather than the nurturing mother-hen image that would be described by the term *maternalism*.

The 9+9-oriented physician has often been held up as the ideal for medical practice. The good and bad qualities of this style have been particularly difficult for physicians to fully understand. During testing of groups of physicians regarding the soundest solutions to medical dilemmas, the 9+9 leadership style is consistently ranked second only to the 9,9 medical style. This would seem to suggest that it is perceived as the second best way to practice medicine. However, another phenomenon seen during our seminars seems to challenge this assumption. In an analysis of actual practice style, the participants seldom rank 9+9 that high. More importantly, when intergroup exchange about style occurs in training seminars, the dislike of dealing with paternalistic physicians always seems to come up.

The dangers inherent in this approach to medical care are subtle, but when unrecognized they can lead the physician into a highly vulnerable situation, compromising quality. This physician is not free of human error, and when he or she takes full responsibility for the medical outcome that results, a lawsuit may be the response of the patient. Certain characteristics of this style can actually create difficult patients, and that never improves the quality of care.

Motivation

The positive motivation for this style, whether conscious or not, is to gain admiration and adulation through giving patients the benefits of one's knowledge, experience, and guidance. A large amount of gratification comes from sharing one's wisdom for the benefit of others. When patients meet the paternalist physician's expectations by complying with instructions, the patients are rewarded by the physician's obvious approval. The patients in turn are expected to appreciate the help and guidance provided to them.

The negative motivational force behind this style is fear of not trying hard enough and being repudiated. This physician feels threatened when patients substitute their own wills and disregard what they have been told. When they resist directions and counsel, they are viewed as disloyal and may be deemed unworthy of further help. The comment, "You work your heart out and the patients don't appreciate it," characterizes this physician's response to a noncompliant patient who does not recognize the physician's sacrifice.

The natural tendency has always been for patients to remain dependent by yielding to the physician's wishes. Because tradition has supported this attitude, patients have been discouraged from growing and developing toward independence of thought, judgment, convictions, and, ultimately, self-care. In the long run, this has a significant negative impact on public health and utilization of a medical resource that is declining.

The 9+9-Oriented Physician-Patient Relationship

Providing Patient Care

As this particular Grid style is a unique combination of 1,9 and 9,1 leadership elements, it stands to reason that this style is characterized by its own special brand of leadership. Without reviewing the various aspects of the 1,9- and 9,1-oriented physicians, as those are well described in previous chapters, this discussion will limit itself to the unique and sometimes subtle ways that the paternalist behaves in each of the six elements of leadership and how this behavior impacts the physician-patient relationship.

Communication. When the 9+9-oriented physician makes a diagnosis and clarifies a treatment plan with the patient, adequate attention is applied to the medical expertise behind the decision. The physician is knowledgeable and an aura of authority is assumed to bolster the patient's confidence. The discussion is likely to convey warmth and caring, and the patient is given adequate time to assimilate the new information. Questions are asked to ensure full understanding before moving on to new information. On the surface, it seems communication could not be better. The difficulty is that this physician has already determined the "right way to go" so that communication really just becomes a strategy to make sure that the patient has been completely won over.

Like a coaching model, paternalism encompasses not only applying rules

69

and regulations, but seeing that they are followed. This physician is quick to compliment patients, seeing his or her power over the patient as great enough to ensure future "good boy" or "good girl" behavior. If the rules are not followed, then the patient learns the physician's displeasure at once, again with the assumption that the physician's reprimand is enough to alter the patient's behavior.

The easiest way to envision the communication that occurs between a 9+9-oriented physician and the patient is to picture a parent trying to control an unruly child. The socialization required of children is for their own good. And so it goes for patients. It is an age-old approach to move children safely into their adulthood and just as age-old an approach to get patients who have been considered childlike and helpless to accept medical care. The difficulty is that children grow up and parents who continue to use this manner of communication with their adult children face rebellion.

We have entered an era in which patients, for a variety of reasons, are moving to a level of greater maturity and independence. The 9+9-oriented physician has not recognized this shift and attempts to keep patients in the child role. This effort becomes obvious to any well-educated or perceptive patient. If the physician is not capable of treating the patient as an adult, hostility may result from the communication style itself.

Establishing patient expectations. Patients sense that the paternalistic physician believes he or she has their own best interests in mind. This is what makes it so hard for patients to resist the strong recommendations of the physician. In many cases, patients adopt the physician's expectations, yet they may resent being treated like children, without wills of their own. The potential for patient resentment to build up is greater under this orientation than any other. Because some patients want to exercise independent thinking but are "not allowed" to do so, they feel forced to accept this parent figure's assertions as absolutely true. As the patients' expectations are not personally owned, they remain shallow, yet they place a burden on the physician because they carry the illusion of a guarantee of perfect outcome.

All the opportunities from which the patients might have gained deeper insight into the real medical situation are blocked in advance by the 9+9 communication style. For some patients, being treated in this paternalistic manner is resented even more than being forced into treatment by a 9,1-oriented physician. The reason is that a patient can fight back when being pushed around by a 9,1-oriented physician; however, to fight back against a paternalist is to fight against what seems to be one's own best interest. Therefore, patients allow the one-way dialogue, even though resentment is stored up as long as it cannot be expressed.

If patients are not willing to let the physician set their expectations, they may abandon medical care completely, especially if resentment has reached a high level. Once out of the system these patients are unlikely to return for fear of getting trapped in the same untenable situation again. If this feeling is strong enough, the opportunity to treat the patient is lost and what is sadder still is that these often intelligent, independent-thinking patients would have been willing participants in 9,9 decision making if only a different communication approach had been used.

Acquiring Knowledge. Because the 9+9-oriented physician feels an obligation to tell people what to do, to guide their actions, and to counsel them, much inquiry is focused on gathering information and ensuring that everything is going according to the physician's expectations. It may be direct in the sense of asking for reports or checking charts, but more often the questions are intended to let patients know what is wanted of them. This may even border on manipulation. The paternalist relies on questions as a primary teaching tool to determine if patients can respond correctly. If so, the lesson has been learned; if not, further instructions are needed. Listening skills are high, but they are used as often to be sure that goals are met as to gain new information.

There is a high degree of "need to know" for this physician, because he or she cannot afford to be wrong. Written medical-technical information is heavily relied upon to keep informed, but no need is perceived to gain knowledge related to communication or other leadership skills, as these are already assumed to be at their highest level of development.

Rules and regulations may also be well rehearsed if they are considered relevant. No detail of how the hospital functions is so small that it can be skipped over, because the 9+9-oriented physician assumes at least partial responsibility for everybody employed there.

Assessing the patient's needs. The assessment of a patient's needs can be accurate on the part of this physician. However, because this particular orientation has elements of two basic Grid styles, its assessment is unique. The 9,1-oriented direction sees to it that the patient accepts this physician's assumption of what is needed in medical terms and does not make a mistake in follow-up. The 1,9-oriented aspect assesses the patient's human needs, offering warmth and affection, or whatever else may be needed, in exchange for acceptance of the physician's guidance.

The paternalistic orientation is significant in that it "locks" reluctant patients in, obligating them to accept treatment, even though they may prefer not to do so. The physician insists that the patient-accept care, bypassing a sound patient understanding of why — and yet not in a coercive, hard-sell way either. Rather, it is in the sense of "Father knows best," or "You must take this for your own good." The patient's needs are met as long as the physician is correct in the assumptions made.

Decision Making. When it comes to decisions, this physician has strong beliefs and advocates them intensely, often with an overtone of moralism, with *shoulds, should nots, oughts,* and *must nots.* When patients admire and respect the convictions the physician embraces, the adulation that this physician needs is likely to follow.

Paternalistic physicians see themselves as the sole medical decision makers, and the patient's responsibility is compliance. Decisions are not barked out as commands. Rather, once having decided what a patient should do, teaching, coaching, and counseling are used to help the patient fully understand and accept the recommendation. The physician's approach may vary, but the result is that the patient learns in an imitative or a rote way to do whatever has been taught. This approach forces the patient to check back rather than to operate on personal initiative. The patient fulfills the physician's expectation, and because the patient's role in decision making has been removed, the physician is responsible for a perfect outcome.

Level of responsibility. Possibly the most significant result of 9+9 decision making is the removal of patient responsibility. The problem this creates is clear when the physician is heard to say, "My patients are reluctant to accept responsibility. They are bright and capable, with plenty of know-how, but they can't keep out of trouble. They won't take the ball and run. It is difficult to see how they will ever get well." What the physician fails to realize is that his or her patients are trying to please the physician, but without personal responsibility they find little motivation to exercise initiative on their own.

When the imperfections of medicine bring injury, the patient feels disillusioned and abandoned. If the patient had wanted to share responsibility and feels like a fool for having given the physician permission to provide a therapy or a treatment that the patient did not understand, hatred and a desire for revenge may replace the love once felt. This is an emotionally wrenching and destructive process that could have been avoided if this level of responsibility had not been unnecessarily shouldered by the physician.

Initiative. Once decisions are made, the 9+9-oriented physician exercises strong initiative until the patients can be trusted to obey and follow through in a correct manner. When anything out of the ordinary arises, the physician insists that patients check back rather than acting on their own. With good outcomes, these patients are happy. Some will always prefer to follow and be told what to do. The physician, of course, assumes that this is sound medicine. After all, "Patients really don't have the ability to think for themselves, not when medical issues are concerned."

In emergencies, the 9+9 approach is generally efficient: 9,1 aggressive, straightforward efforts to initiate actions that solve problems are balanced with

1,9 recaps of why "we had to respond in this way for your own good." The patient is expected to understand and accept the explanation.

Conflict Resolution

Dealing with patient objections. The 9+9-oriented physician expects patients to object now and then, much as children who do not understand the adult world. This physician sees objections as an opportunity to educate and mold the patient into a "better complier." However, from the patient's perspective, the objection is never sincerely dealt with, let alone resolved.

Avoiding conflict. The first step is always to avoid conflict by maintaining control. That can be accomplished by positive reinforcement of compliance. Once patients come to expect and feel secure with praise and compliments, the physician can withhold the positive strokes as an indication of displeasure. If this does not work and patients continue to resist or to exhibit poor compliance, the physician may reprimand, letting the patients know that bad behavior has been exhibited and that poor health is their own fault. The physician then repeats what is wanted, possibly using the exact same words of explanation, as if the patients were too dull to comprehend what was said the first time. Praise is then offered in anticipation that compliance will be forthcoming. This can become downright patronizing.

Handling patient conflict. One way to reduce conflict is to divert attention from disagreement by changing the subject or placing the problem in an alternative context. Shifting contexts keeps this physician from ever having to admit being wrong. It also lets the patient yield without being made to feel guilty for disagreeing.

Handling medical team conflict. When a paternalistic solution is applied to conflicts involving members of the medical team, a new problem arises. The physician sees the solution as simple: "You two get in a room and solve this problem." Even though this approach is designed to eliminate the conflict, it also rests on the assumption that those who are in conflict can resolve their disagreement by an act of will. This, of course, is rarely true, even though the physician's feeling of control is fully restored when the team members express appreciation and gratitude for all the physician has done to help them resolve their differences. Controlling members of the medical team is also done through reward and punishment. This is the model of paternalistic child-rearing extended into the hospital setting.

When conflict persists. When conflict remains unresolved and control cannot be reestablished, the patient may be disowned. This solution is what underlies the statement, "I can't believe it. Think of all I've done for that patient." Taking the role of the martyr, the physician rejects the ungrateful patient. Once a break in the physician-patient relationship occurs, it is likely to be permanent, with little the patient can do to get back in the good graces of the physician.

On the grand scale. Against a background of what had appeared to be a stable and long-enduring tradition, waves of resentment and retaliation have recently broken out against the field of medicine. There has been a shift from compliant acceptance to a defiant patient and public retaliation. The conflict that plagues medicine as a whole may be the direct result of 9+9 leadership unable to adapt in a changing society.

Medical care that discourages, if not rejects, the thinking and capabilities of people generates frustration, resistance, and alienation. These feelings are difficult to express directly to a physician whose fatherly concerns seem to have the best interests of the patient in mind. As a result, reactions to felt indignities may be swallowed and bottled up for a time, but they are there. By masking what is at times a seething resentment and unrest, the patient gives the appearance of docility and devotion, even though the tension under these circumstances is so great that even a minor irritation can trigger an eruption of vitriolic reactions.

One psychological formula for concocting hate consists of arousing resentment under conditions of dependency. Because this situation and the conflicts that ensue cannot be resolved within the 9+9 medical system, objections to the paternalistic model of medical care tend to be fought out in a courtroom, much to the amazement of the paternalistic physician. It is not uncommon to hear this physician say, "I can't believe it. She was my favorite patient. She brought me flowers. I did everything possible. Everybody gets complications. If this patient is taking doctors to court, then we're in real trouble." Physicians seldom recognize that the traditional approach to medicine and the paternalistic physician have set the whole situation up. Just like children grow up, so has the current population of patients; if physicians continue to treat them like children, they will leave home, or worse, they will burn the house down.

Critique and Feedback. The 9+9-oriented physician usually shuts off feedback from patients and even other members of the medical team. This may masquerade as humility, but negative comments would suggest a weakness, and the paternalistic physician takes pride in his or her perceived infallibility. Personal feedback goes in one direction, from the physician down, because everyone else is below the physician. Patients and medical team members understand this and limit their reactions to weaker or stronger applause. However, if "father knows best," little or nothing can be learned from children;

therefore, everyone is expected to take a "be seen and not heard" orientation, despite the need for criticism.

A special problem occurs around the issue of informed consent.

Informed consent. To the 9+9-oriented physician, this special type of critique and feedback requires lecture-style education. This physician may be an excellent traditional teacher, meaning he or she delivers information well. The patient comes away from the interview having heard about the procedures suggested, the risks and the benefits, how long a hospitalization will be required, what the recovery time will be, what restrictions on activity will be necessary, and what the procedure will cost. The difficulty is that too often the tone is one of unrealistic expectations and no real shared responsibility. Rather than making informed consent a type of pre-critique through which the patient, as an essential member of the team, irons out problems of understanding and clarifies the roles that will lead toward their mutual goals, the signature on the hospital form is simply permission to carry out treatment prescribed by the physician. The power of this physician's control over the patient does not come through informed consent contracts; it comes through the emotional dependency that has been created. The possibility of less than a perfect outcome seldom comes up before the signature is in place on the consent form.

After care has been delivered, this physician feels no reluctance in giving feedback to patients. It is the physician's obligation to pass on to the patients whatever they need to know for their own good. Then they can benefit from the wisdom and guidance that has been offered them.

For all of this physician's good qualities, the inability to use active listening and to change, based on evaluating the feedback of others, limits this individual's ability to practice truly excellent medicine.

New and Established Patients

The 9+9 approach has a tendency to draw a particular type of patient. The office is warm and inviting. He or she is very likely to have a maternalistic nurse, one who will nurture, to complement the need of the physician to father the patients. New patients are thoroughly evaluated, and after adequate information is gathered, the physician determines a diagnosis that will direct the patient's care from that point forward. Established patients tend to be those who have been successfully treated in the past and who have established a workable relationship with this physician. For patients who have conceded self-responsibility because the field of medicine is too complex, the paternalistic physician is their savior. This attitude engenders a great deal of follow-up business for the physician. This physician's practice may thrive, as it has been one of the most common practice styles handed down from a tradition that made Marcus Welby a household name.

Coping with the Busy Practice

The physician with a 9+9 orientation is generally quite busy, occasionally complaining of the requirements that the field of medicine places on a caring, concerned physician. The waiting room of this physician is likely to be packed. Making the patients wait is not intentional but is considered an inevitable part of meeting all the patients' needs. Because the wait reflects the physician's perception of quality patient care, the physician accepts patient criticism in this area and genuinely apologizes for any inconvenience that has been caused. Because patients tend to relate to this physician as to a father, they are often forgiving. However, expectations subconsciously grow higher and higher when any sacrifice is made in an attempt to maintain harmony.

The difficulty with the busy practice that this physician has established is that it causes fatigue and stress, elements contributing to physician error. All physicians are human, and this is true for the 9+9-oriented physician as well. However, the relationship that this physician establishes with patients precludes human error.

Having a busy practice is also positive reinforcement for the behavior patterns that this physician has come to accept as optimal medical care. This subtle self-deception provides an obstacle in understanding the benefits to change.

Scheduling and Time Management. Within this physician's busy practice, scheduling and time management are simply parts of a highly evolved organizational system. "I think out in advance what it is that needs to be achieved and how to go about it, and then I seek to involve others in independently coming to the same conclusion."

"I organize all aspects of medical care and see that my patients appreciate my efforts."

The Hospital. "In the hospital, I discuss what needs to be done to the point where nurses and other members of the medical team come to see it my way. I reward their efforts and withhold praise or give reprimands to those who do not cooperate. When people balk, I hold out the promise of reward for renewed effort to do it right. I am dedicated to my hospital."

"I rely on and utilize those whose loyalty I can depend on."

Expenses. "Medical practice will always be monetarily rewarding. My expenses are considered high by many people's standards, but I demand the best for my patients and that costs a little extra."

Continuing Education. "Continuing medical education seminars are a farce. I maintain my clinical expertise by reading, attending morbidity and mortality conferences and grand rounds, preparing myself to educate resident staff, and participating in nursing in-service. This helps me not only to keep clinically on top of the latest literature but also to be reassured that house staff and nurses meet my high standards of excellence."

Self-Evaluation. "I evaluate myself through observing my patients and members of the medical team. If I can keep them on the straight-and-narrow track, then I know that I am doing my job. When patients comply and the medical team moves ever closer to excellence, I have all the self-evaluation I need."

Recognizing 9+9 Behavior

Before moving on to patient reactions to a 9+9 Grid style, some familiar words and phrases are good indicators of this leadership style:

Benevolent dictator
Condescending
Constantly gives advice
Discharges obligations
Expects blind loyalty
Graciously demanding
Jealously guards prerogatives
Leader of the flock
Leads by inspirational zeal
Makes those who disagree feel guilty
Martyr
Moralistic
Patronizing
Perfectionist
Preachy
Prescriptive
Self-righteous
Stands for the "virtues"
Tolerates private disagreement but resents public challenge

Patient Reactions Based On Grid Styles

Patient reactions to the 9+9 style may vary based on the patient's response to the cycle of praise and reprimand that this physician exhibits. The specific challenges that face the paternalistic physician are described in the following analysis of each patient style.

9,1

When the 9+9-oriented physician establishes a relationship with a 9,1-oriented patient, war or resignation is the likely outcome. If the patient attacks, the battle is much more subtle than that which would be waged against a 9,1-oriented physician. Because 9+9-oriented physicians feel genuine concern about meeting the needs of their patients, the physician's efforts to change the patient tend to be more persistent than in the 9,1 approach. If the patient is unyielding, the stress of the situation may push the physician into a back-up style that precludes healthy resolution of the conflict.

The 9,1 back-up style is confrontational, indicating that the patient is free to leave, much as an insulting adolescent may be psychologically abandoned by a disenchanted parent. The intent of a 1,9 back-up would be to try to win the patient's affection at all costs. Another possibility would be 1,1 resignation, when it becomes clear that this obstinate patient cannot be won over.

The reason that the 9,1 orientation is so difficult for this physician is that he or she is the most likely to be genuinely insulted by the patronizing attitude that conveys, "This patient couldn't possibly know what is wrong medically." This 9+9 approach may force the angry patient into a deliberately unhelpful role and into the courtroom to prove this physician wrong in cases of a less-than-perfect outcome.

1,9

The 1,9-oriented patient represents the other end of the spectrum, because he or she is automatically attracted to the 9+9 style. This patient is the child who wants to be loved and who has conceded any sense of self-responsibility for medical knowledge. The danger is that this patient gladly gives up all responsibility for health to the paternalistic physician, who is happy to accept it. All is well as long as the outcome is good and the patient is never disillusioned. But when this patient is let down by this father figure, the disappointment is overwhelming, and there is an overreaction to the poor outcome, which is seen as an issue of quality. The next step may be that this patient, who brought the physician a present on his or her birthday, has sued.

1,1

Patients who are 1,1 oriented are difficult for any physician to move to an attitude that allows for excellent medical care, but the 9+9-oriented physician has a fairly good chance of delivering appropriate care to these patients because they fit the physician's assumptions. These patients truly are somewhat helpless within the system. The conflict that will occur between this patient and the 9+9-oriented physician is based on the fact that this patient will not admire, revere, or even be particularly loyal to this physician, for whom these responses are essential for career satisfaction. The relationship may be enduring as long as the patient is relatively silent, accepting of the care, and not obviously unimpressed. Because these physicians are caring, they are quite capable of determining the fundamental medical needs of the burned-out patient, much like a veterinarian faced with a dog or a cat that is unable to speak. The limitations of communication are accepted, and care is rendered within those limitations.

The 9+9-oriented physician is unlikely to improve the quality of care that is possible by moving this patient to a point of self-responsibility, at which point the cycle of ignoring medical advice until a crisis arises could end. The 1,1-oriented patient attitude is affirmed by the nurturing paternalistic care this physician is so comfortable in providing. The patronizing, "Now, now, that's a good patient" may be heard as praise, when the patient has simply taken a pill. The reprimand of "Now, you should know better than that" is met with a blank stare, which the physician prefers to ignore. Because the physician's assumption is that the patient would not be able to act independently, educating the patient in the concept of preventative medicine is completely neglected, and an opportunity for higher quality care is missed.

5,5

The 5,5-oriented, middle-of-the-road patient seeking a successful physician with a good reputation will often end up in a 9+9-oriented physician's office. These patients who come to admire this physician will tell everyone they know how lucky they are to be receiving such excellent care. This is one of the primary sources of encouragement for 9+9 behavior in a physician. The 5,5-oriented patient is usually rewarded by the paternalistic physician, who probes personal desires and provides sound feedback. Riding on an excellent reputation, this physician has little difficulty convincing the patient that the services that are recommended will be appropriate and will meet that individual's needs for a therapy that has been proven effective and has been acclaimed by their family and friends.

The difficulty with 5,5-oriented patients is that they perpetually fear being taken advantage of, and they are embarrassed by the criticism that inevitably follows slow compliance on their part. This situation can occur frequently, as these patients are not striving for genuine self-responsibility, but rather for doing what the "in" crowd is doing and avoiding any discomfort. Even though these patients can tell that the physician is caring, the embarrassment they feel after a reprimand may be harbored for quite some time as resentment. If this feeling is perpetuated, the physician may be starting a time bomb ticking, all with quite good intentions.

9,9

Patients who are 9,9 oriented approach the 9+9-oriented physician with an unusual understanding of what this unique physician-patient interaction is all about. The 9+9-oriented physician listens, provides sound medical advice, and shows a genuine concern for the human needs of the patient who sits before him or her. The difficulty arises when this physician demonstrates, at some point in the interview, that enough information has been gathered and that the necessary decisions have been made. All that remains is to convince the patient to comply, to become a loyal follower, and to show the appropriate appreciation.

These patients demand some level of self-responsibility and will question the physician at points of disagreement about patient need or where the patient's information is not in line with the medical advice the physician has rendered. This patient is concerned about the feelings of the physician but does not want to be treated as a child. If the physician tries to bypass these questions as unimportant — "After all, you're only the patient and I am the doctor"- then the patient becomes frustrated. Even though the physician can provide both the emotional feedback and intellectual information required by this patient, he or she responds negatively to spoon-feeding. This patient finds the parent-like approach of this physician unappealing and may abandon the physician to continue a search for another physician who treats patients like adults and like equals.

If the 9,9-oriented patient's questioning is misinterpreted by the physician and this physician begins to feel that the patient is not only disloyal but disrespectful, it may be the physician who abandons the patient. In either event, the potential for two individuals very well equipped to establish a physician-patient relationship and to take full advantage of the medical expertise that is present will be lost, and poor-quality medical care may result.

Summary

The 9+9-oriented physician is a difficult one to evaluate because the weaknesses in the style are subtle. The issue of self-deception creeps into this style because paternalists believe they are providing the best medical care. The 9+9-oriented physician is hard working, genuinely concerned, and usually considered to be a good teacher. This physician feels almost inspired to be a physician and is dedicated to meeting the needs of patients. The difficulty arises when this benevolent dictator feels compelled to give advice to those who are not asking for it in a moralistic or self-righteous way and demands blind loyalty. If the advice is rejected, the physician may feel martyred, being shocked when those who have received so much good care or good advice are ungrateful.

The 9+9-oriented physician may have many of the qualities that lead to excellent medical care, but the one recurring difficulty this physician faces is the creation of children out of patients. This condescending attitude may lead patients to resentments that surface whenever medical care falls short of perfection.

The overall consequences of the 9+9 orientation are a restriction on personal growth for the physician and a limitation on self-responsibility for the patient. Medical team members suffer under this orientation, and subordinate members of the team (nurses in particular) are quick to point out that this type of physician is present in large numbers in every hospital across the country. Under the best of circumstances, the system can function, yet the volatile relationships that often evolve between a parent and child can allow patient trust and loyalty to be replaced by resentment and even revenge. This may be one of the most subtle yet pervasive quality issues in American medical care.

Chapter Seven

1,1 MEDICAL CARE: LEARNING THE ART OF SURVIVAL

"Well, do you think we ought to call the duck in from home?" Velma asked with a laugh. "Or do you think we ought to just let the patient take her own X-rays?" Looking at the call schedule from the ER, there didn't seem to be a choice.

"Well, I'm not sure which would be better," chuckled Nancy. "I'm going to see if I can get transferred to another floor before he comes in. I don't think I can handle working with him. I was just reading about one of his patients the other day."

"Yeah, first X-rays; then it's off to the CAT scan," Velma snickered.

Just then Dr. Thompson walked in, "Do I hear what you two are talking about? Donald Bill was reading X-rays before you were even born. You have no idea what an illustrious career he has had. He trained at Northwestern University back when Chicago had the best medical program around and then went on to do a surgical residency. He was an accomplished surgeon before going into radiology, and when he came back to this town, he really knocked them on their ear. You should have seen him — dramatic, handsome. He started our department here. Yeah, he had the world by the tail. The only criticism you can really make of him now is that he may be trying to hang on a little too long, but that man can read X-rays in his sleep. So let's not hear all of this joking. Let's give the man a little respect."

"Oh, I'm sorry, Dr. Thompson. I really didn't mean anything." Apologizing as she left the room, Velma went back to ready the patient for transfer to X-ray. She winked at Nancy as she headed down the hall, mumbling "quack, quack."

Nancy couldn't help but laugh. She looked up at Dr. Thompson, who was shaking his head in disgust to hide the fact that he, too, found it hard not to smile. "Dr. Thompson, we're just kidding. You know the du-, I mean Dr. Bill is getting a little nearsighted and keeps walking in the wrong room, so it's just a little extra work for us to try to keep things straightened out. We really didn't mean anything by our jokes."

The patient was suffering from right upper quadrant abdominal pain and had been vomiting. She seemed a bit angry, as it was her second trip to the ER, and she really didn't have much to say. She just hoped that the doctors knew what was best for her.

Just then Dr. Bill rolled into the ER with a stack of newspapers and crossword puzzles to pass the time until the techs had taken the films. Dr. Bill always stayed in the ER until the X-rays were complete, occasionally talking to the family. His presence gave the appearance of extreme concern. Yet the nurses knew that there would be no predicting when he would decide it was time to read the films, or if he would identify a problem that did not exist or ignore an obvious one. As other physicians moved in and out of the ER, Dr. Bill always said "Hello," criticized the increased competition and the new techniques that "aren't worth a damn anyway," and rattled on about the days when he was reading all of the films single-handedly during World War II.

When the doctors' lounge cleared, Dr. Bill would stay in the same chair, staring at the wall, his intent gaze broken only by occasional glances at the crossword puzzle, which remained unfinished in his lap. He did not initiate conversations with the nurses but was quick to reply to any questions. Even though he came in from home, it was common for him to be in the hospital several hours once he'd been called in.

Something was wrong with Dr. Bill besides his failing eyesight, shortened memory, and increasing years. It was as if he were angry at the world, new techniques, new competition, hospital rules and regulations, and the recent lawsuits that had prompted the hospital credentials committee to suggest his retirement. There was also a certain lack of energy in this anger. His agitation had no real focus and no real origin that you could put your finger on. Dr. Bill had indeed been one of the best physicians of his time, but his time had passed. He knew it, yet financial obligations forced him to continue to trudge through the routine that kept him just busy enough to stay employed by the hospital's department of radiology.

Suddenly Dr. Bill sat up, took a deep breath, walked to the front desk, and said, "Let's find out what this lady has." The nurse looked up, frowned, and followed Dr. Bill down the hall. Nancy glanced over to Velma, who was carefully slipping into another patient room to avoid being a part of whatever was to follow. Dr. Bill went to the reading room and Nancy got the patient, who was now pale and shocky. The X-ray tech, who had only worked there a few weeks, explained what tests had been done: a flat plate, a KUB, and an ultrasound of the abdomen and pelvis. Dr. Bill thought he saw a cyst of the ovary.

"There's the problem. She probably has a ruptured cyst and is bleeding. That would cause her referral pain: blood under the diaphragm. Let's get a CAT scan to take a better look."

With confirmation from the CAT scan, Dr. Bill returned to the ER with a look of confidence. "Well, Thompson, you got the right tests; that ultrasound solved the dilemma. She has a right ovarian cyst. Looks like fluid in the cul-de-sac, too. She's probably bleeding. Just to be sure, I did a scan and it's there. Everything else is normal."

Dr. Thompson frowned and turned away. "Thanks, Don." He looked at Dr. Pointer, the surgical resident. "Well, that's kind of an expensive pelvic exam."

Pointer replied sharply, "She doesn't have a pelvic mass. CAT scans aren't any good in the pelvis anyway. It's just an artifact. I want to know if she has air under the diaphragm."

"Well, you can't tell that by a pelvic, and Dr. Bill says she's normal."

Pointer was taking the patient's pulse. "She's about to go off, Doctor."

"Obviously, she's in shock. We're just wasting our time here."

They quickly moved her to the OR and upon opening her abdomen, emptied over one liter of fresh blood from the wound, followed by large clots. Dr. Thompson had also done a pelvic and used his clinical judgment to make a midline incision, even though the patient had requested a Pfannenstiel.

It didn't take long to find the perforated duodenal ulcer.

"This patient had to have air under the diaphragm," barked Dr. Pointer. He called for the films and just as he suspected, the area of the diaphragm was cut off the top of the film. "You can't read that. This is ridiculous." The surgeons quickly finished the case. Neither said anything other than the usual short commands — "Suture, Kelly, scissors."

Dr. Pointer walked out of the operating room with a pale expression and said, "How can you let that turkey get away with that?" Dr. Thompson looked up, shook his head, and said nothing. Dr. Pointer said, "Well, I'm reporting this. This is ridiculous. That patient spent too much time in X-ray and for what? I don't understand why he's still on staff."

Dr. Thompson looked up and said, "Well, that's why you're a resident. You still have a lot to learn."

When the case came up for review, Dr. Thompson came to Dr. Bill's rescue. He was already feeling the boredom of a routine, repetitive approach to patient care and was beginning to understand the temptation to fall behind.

Dr. Pointer, a young, idealistic physician, had not learned to tolerate the lack of concern or the deficient skills that now characterized Dr. Bill. He felt it was his moral duty to go after Dr. Bill, and all it did was create barriers for himself. He was accused of being a witch hunter — young, incompetent, undertrained physician trying to flex his tender muscles.

Dr. Bill continued to practice, finally threatening the hospital with a lawsuit on the grounds that they were trying to remove his ability to provide himself a livelihood. He never understood why the entire medical system seemed to turn on him after all he had done to advance medicine in his long, illustrious career.

General Characteristics of the 1,1-Orientation to Medicine

The physician who has adopted a 1,1-oriented philosophy is committed neither to mastering the medical complexities of practice nor to meeting human needs. This physician has turned inward, and survival within the medical system has become the only concern.

The 1,1 leadership pattern is located in the lower left corner of the Grid. The physician experiences little or no contradiction between medical achievement and the needs of people, because concern for both is so low. Being more or less "out of it" while remaining in practice, the physician expects little and little is given. Enthusiasm for medical care has disappeared, but practice is still a requirement to meet financial obligations.

Motivation

The positive motivation in a 1,1 orientation is to exert the minimum effort to "hang on" and "remain in the system." Appearing occupied and seeming to be concentrating on some activity are well practiced in order to direct attention of peers away from oneself. The degree to which the 1,1-oriented physician can remain passive and unnoticed and still survive is governed by the minimum others are prepared to tolerate. The medical system has been hesitant to "point fingers" and criticize any physician, even when chart reviews and audit committees indicate that some individuals have fallen into a 1,1 pattern of practice.

The negative motivation of physicians with a 1,1 orientation is to avoid financial disaster. This means taking whatever steps are necessary to conceal from patients, and frequently even from themselves, the boredom and fatigue that might lead to a lost patient or recognition that they have burned out.

It is impossible for this physician to remain entirely invisible, although the philosophy of "see no evil, speak no evil, and hear no evil" becomes this physician's motto. The physician hopes to pass through the last years of practice leaving no permanent mark or scars that cannot be recovered from. However, the medical profession may have already left its mark on this physician by "pushing the physician past the breaking point" or merely letting the physician drift from some other more preferable Grid style into the 1,1 corner, with the comment, "Oh well, it won't be long until he (or she) retires."

The 1,1-Oriented Physician-Patient Relationship

The notion of a person in the medical context having both a low concern for patients and a low concern for maintaining medical expertise may at first glance seem improbable. Yet everyone knows someone who has adopted this orientation. These individuals make no dramatic splash, and it is unlikely that as one of their peers you have really gotten to know them. The problems that face

1,1-oriented physicians and the ones that they create can be examined by looking at the various aspects of the 1,1 medical practice.

Providing Patient Care

The 1,1 attitude promotes little involvement and participation by the patient or the team providing medical care. Rather than mutual problem solving, the attitude tends to be: "Patients come to me for what I offer. If they don't, there's nothing I can do about it. I provide whatever information I have. That's my job." This attitude leaves the rest of the medical team devoid of leadership and faced with the challenge of having to pursue a one-sided conversation.

Communication. Interacting with a 1,1-oriented physician is an odd experience. The physician sits down and speaks briefly, with little enthusiasm. The patient has an eerie feeling that a prerecorded announcement is being played but nevertheless listens, hoping to glean something from the discussion. The comments may be totally unrelated to the symptoms presented; at the very least, it soon becomes obvious that a precise answer will not be forthcoming — this machine is simply not equipped to give one. This physician can get away with this sort of physician-patient encounter because the patients often assume that they themselves are confused.

Listening that is 1,1 oriented is generally inattentive, as the physician is neither emotionally involved with the treatment nor interested in the personal encounter that is taking place. The physician may even daydream as he or she recites the well-memorized diagnosis and treatment plan that this patient has fallen into. If the patient seems unready to proceed with the treatment, the physician conveys disapproval, yet the underlying attitude is, "Well, this one's gone down the drain, there's nothing more to discuss." Rather than moving forward in a sound manner to bring the patient to understanding, the physician terminates the interview.

Interruption is taken as another sign that the patient is uninterested in the treatment plan, but all is not lost because of the free time that the patient's early departure provides. While dealing perfunctorily with the interruption, this physician is mentally putting on a coat and walking out the door. "At least that one didn't take long; maybe I can get away early."

The patient may be questioning the medical treatment in order to understand it better, but the physician will not risk convincing the patient to participate if there are any questions at all. Giving up is a self-fulfilling prophecy, but in a way it protects the physician from those patients who might ultimately question outcomes. The decreased number of patients is rationalized as part of the new competition, but at a subconscious level this physician has learned that having fewer patients is a necessity to stay hidden and unchallenged.

Establishing patient expectations. The 1,1-oriented physician avoids anything that might lead to the development of positive expectations. This physician sets strict boundaries as to what the patient can reasonably anticipate and, in this way, avoids having to explain or rationalize in order to appease a disappointed patient.

This approach to setting expectations is demonstrated in the following conversation:

Physician: Anything else?
Patient: Yes, there is. I've heard they're coming out with some new treatments. Advances seem to be just around the corner these days. Maybe we should wait awhile.
Physician: That's up to you.
Patient: But what do you think the prospects are for something that could be better for me?
Physician: I don't know of any treatments that are better.
Patient: Well, what do you think?
Physician: I just told you what the risks and benefits of your treatment are. But if you want to wait, it's your life.
Patient: No, I'm sure you're right.

The patient cannot exactly look back on this experience and say, "I was sold a bill of goods." The patient made the final decision not to consider alternatives, and that is the protection that allows this type of physician to continue in practice.

Acquiring Knowledge. This physician pursues knowledge only to the degree that it is necessary to avoid appearing ill informed or revealing an ignorance of new medical technology. When asked a question, the physician does not admit to lack of knowledge but responds, "I'll check," yet never finds the time. This response deters the criticism that would come from saying, "I don't know," and it relieves the tensions that peers inevitably feel when faced with this type of physician.

The physician with a predominantly 1,1 attitude is unlikely to gain more than casual understanding of new medical techniques. If questioned closely about the medical therapy, the physician might reply, "These are the general details. It's hard for anyone to keep up with the technical complexity nowadays. I'd be happy to loan you my textbook on it if you need more information." The most this physician can be expected to do during the patient-physician interview is to reach for a book to show pictures and charts or read from a product insert or the PDR.

Assessing the patient's needs. The normal practice for this physician is to bypass anything approaching a needs analysis. Discussion is rarely initiated about how a treatment may impact the individual's personal life, let alone about the illness that brought the patient to the physician in the first place. The physician justifies this approach by saying, "Doing more than considering the basic facts is a waste of effort. There is no sense in trying to probe what the patient is thinking. If patients didn't want what I have to offer, they wouldn't have come to me as their physician."

Decision Making. The 1,1-oriented physician is noncommittal and reticent, avoiding decisions whenever possible. However, when faced with a situation that demands a decision, this physician tends to sidestep. If the question is "What do you think?" the answer is evasive. If a more detailed question requires a yes or no decision, the reply will usually be "perhaps" or "maybe." If an opinion is voiced, the reply may be, "I guess you're right." Yet you get the feeling that no decision has really been made and that the physician, given time, will allow a situation to take its own course or kind of ferment until other care providers have had a chance to step in and solve the problem.

Physicians who are 1,1 oriented occasionally find themselves in a crisis that is well over their heads. If the opportunity exists, the physician is likely to hand care over to the resident and say, "You're the chief; you're going to be out in practice next year. You ought to be able to handle this sort of problem. Now you get to see what it's really like." However, if there is no resident to turn to, the physician is forced to look inside, and when no answers are forthcoming, the recurrent theme is to leave well enough alone. These physicians will literally turn their backs on the patient as they walk out of the room muttering, "More time is needed. I'll have to think about it." The physician may then corner the charge nurse and ask, "What's the hospital policy? Where is that protocol we developed?" As the physician begins to pore over the information, hoping to find a cookbook remedy to the patient's situation, more time is lost. The task of the consultant, who will eventually come in and try to bail this physician out, becomes ever more difficult.

This physician at times appears to be a good delegator of responsibility. The reality is that it is more like abdication in cases where the physician feels uncomfortable. The rationalization is, "Giving these problems to the nurses and residents helps them grow and creates good learning experiences." This system provides good medical care and protects this physician, as long as nurses and residents are not given tasks that are too difficult. Without significant leadership, a more common outcome is that the entire team falls apart. The astute nurse or resident who is familiar with this physician's abilities inevitably finds some other "understanding" physician willing to come to the rescue. However, if one is not available, the ultimate in poor-quality care is realized and the disaster runs its full course.

Physicians who are 1,1 oriented extol the virtues of teamwork and delegation in their never-ending attempts to effectively remove themselves from the responsibility of decision making. Although the technique has become a requirement for this physician's survival, it is a major barrier to the highly competent teamwork that is a requirement of medical excellence. In the worst case, a wrong diagnosis is made and a wrong treatment is applied.

Level of responsibility. This physician assumes almost no responsibility for discovering the patient's human needs and curing the illness that brings the patient to him or her in the first place. This physician generally migrates to techniques that can be performed by the book or hospital protocol so that the whole process of medical care becomes more of a technical trade than a profession. Patients are not invited to share a level of responsibility, they are not given responsibility for themselves, and the physician certainly is not taking full responsibility for the outcome. Patients who remain with this physician are characteristically confused, but "in an era of such high technology, what else can be expected?"

Initiative. The 1,1-oriented physician is apathetic and is unlikely to develop, much less initiate, any new ideas. The intent is to stand pat on old techniques that have "gotten us through the tough times" in the past and to let things run their course. Any action is passive and unassertive, taken mainly to avoid being conspicuous. These physicians will delegate responsibilities to those in subordinate roles rather than take actions themselves. In extreme circumstances, the physician will transfer the patient to a previously tested and somewhat sympathetic physician who enjoys the referral source and is therefore not critical of this physician's competence.

This physician takes no initiative with regard to understanding what the competition offers. Feeling there is really nothing that can be done about it, he or she is not even motivated to initiate a change as patient numbers drop.

Conflict Resolution

Maintaining neutrality. Maintaining neutrality in the face of conflict has been developed to a fine art by this physician. A grunt is the best reply of all. "Hmmmm" sort of sums it up. Even though true, a reply such as "Don't bug me about this; I really don't care," would give away the game and some might even take it as an affront. But "hmmmm" is a deadener. It leaves the other person with no real way to respond, and often the issue is simply dropped.

Other neutral answers are "I was just reading about that the other day..."; "Yes, I heard something about that..."; "I wasn't actually there..."; "It wasn't really up to me..."; "After all, that's not my specialty..."; and possibly the most popular phrase, "You never asked." The 1,1-oriented physician prefers to avoid the appearance of backing off, and neutrality is not actually defeat. A statement like, "Fine, that's your opinion and you're entitled to that" implies that a physician is also entitled to his or her opinion — right or wrong. The key is to ensure that answers never obligate the physician to any particular course of action. The goal is apparent agreement without explicit commitment: "Whatever..."

Dealing with patient objections. These physicians are experts at steering the conversation along an objection-free path by either ignoring the objection or accepting it. In a sense the conversation becomes disconnected. As far as the physician is concerned, no disagreement exists. In retrospect the physician may say,"Well, the patient just couldn't understand what was going on. I don't really blame him; he was under a lot of stress."

If the patient insists on pursuing an objection, the physician is likely to downplay it by saying, "There is little chance of that problem ever coming up during the treatment." When a patient has specific concerns that need resolution, the physician possesses an infinite variety of neutral answers: "You know, we really can't say"; "I haven't heard any new information on that one"; or "None of us were there when the original studies were done, but here's my recommendation." If the patient persists with an objection, the physician is likely to yield, but if it comes to a real choice between dealing fully with the patient's objection or losing the patient, it is preferable to lose the patient altogether.

Playing games/dishonesty. The 1,1-oriented physician "loses" the disturbing reports about patient care that come from the audit committee and "forgets" to attend the morbidity and mortality conferences that each hospital is obligated to hold. If questions come up about the meeting or the reports, there is always an excuse, making subtle dishonesty an inevitable part of the quest to stay hidden.

The 1,1-oriented physician cannot help but observe members of the medical team occasionally working at cross purposes. By keeping out of the way, even to the point of allowing poor care to be delivered, the physician not only avoids conflict, but stores away evidence that can be used later to convince peers that no one has the right to cast stones. The physician actually watches situations deteriorate so that he or she can forgive the member of the medical team who has made a mistake. Inevitably this medical team member will "go to bat" for the 1,1-oriented physician. The result is an entire unit that accepts far less than medical excellence.

Double-talk. This tactic is extremely useful to this physician, as every medical issue has at least two points of view. The goal here is to speak on both sides of the issue without taking a firm position. Often this type of double-talk can get so far afield that the examples given do not relate to the diagnosis being considered.

"Treatment A may be the best for the reasons that have been given, but, on the other hand, there are strong points on the side of treatment B. It is possible for us to go ahead and do X, but it would be equally as possible for us to do Y." At that point, the physician stops and waits for a reply. Having stated nothing except the obvious, individuals on either side of the controversy may feel the physician has a sympathetic appreciation for their point of view. When one side finally wins out, the physician simply lets the course of action fall in place. If indecision remains, he or she makes a hasty exit on the pretext of the high demand for his or her medical expertise in some other area of the hospital.

Mental walkout. The only way to become free from the burden of unaddressed conflicts and the potential for poor medical outcome is by mentally walking out on the entire situation. If medical team members press for an immediate solution to a medical problem, the 1,1-oriented physician is likely to say, "Everything will work out in a few days. I've seen this situation over and over again." With that, the physician not only leaves the room but resigns the conflict. In time, the situation often does improve because the deteriorating health of the patient inevitably involves a new organ system that requires consultation from other, more competent physicians. As the physician who obtained the consultant, the practitioner may even be able to feign the control that had been voluntarily relinquished a few days prior to the new medical problem.

Critique and Feedback. The 1,1-oriented physician is unlikely to engage in much introspection, because his or her mind is not on the task or the patient at hand. As a result, feedback to others is uncommon and feedback from others has almost no impact.

Informed consent. This physician approaches the informed consent issue in a very matter-of-fact way. It may be little more than a vague question: "Do you feel like going ahead with the treatment?" If the patient wants it, fine; the physician will schedule the surgery or perform the test. In this sense the physician can be viewed as a message carrier, more or less mechanically transmitting the patient's purchase order to the hospital for processing without adding any personal energy. The price is never mentioned spontaneously. Even when the question of cost comes up, this physician may avoid the answer by saying something like, "I'm not certain, but I think you can get that information from the hospital." The physician shifts the responsibility for finding out onto the patient's shoulders.

If the patient's decision is to refuse the treatment, the physician's attitude is, "Well, okay. You can't win them all." Even if the patient showed some initial interest in a proposed treatment, the first mention of the word "no" is accepted as final. "I'm sure you can find someone who will be coerced into providing whatever treatment you want, but it's not me," is the physician's conclusion to the interview.

In the case of a poor outcome, a situation all too familiar to this physician, the only salvation lies in having avoided the creation of false expectations with regard to the treatment plan. Therefore, the physician dismisses the patient who questions the treatment, rather than forcing the signature on an informed consent contract. This attitude does not allow true informed consent for any treatment, but it can give the appearance of such a consent when the patient has requested the procedure and is willing to sign the forms.

This physician is more likely to be successful in a low-risk, primary care setting that requires little more than filling prescriptions, taking throat cultures, and doing routine physical examinations. Such situations usually do not involve life-threatening conditions, and informed consent is easily sidestepped. Unfortunately, physicians who have slipped into the 1,1 orientation, often due to stress, are on occasion operating on hearts, bones, uteruses, bowels, kidneys, and brains. These physicians have rationalized that they, too, can function on autopilot, when in fact the contributions of the patient through informed consent can make a critical difference in whether or not a high-quality outcome is reached.

New and Established Patients

Return patients with chronic problems are likely to be what these physicians rely on for their bread and butter. Because the tradition in medicine is for the patient to seek out the physician, new patients tend to be referrals from established patients who have accepted the 1,1 level of care as inevitable, if somewhat inadequate. The attitude borders on resignation. "Well, why don't you go to Dr. Bill. He's as good as any of them." These physicians do not expect consultation or referral from their peers for obvious reasons. If these physicians happen to be practicing in an area where their specialty is undersupplied, their practice may actually thrive, but that is the exception to the rule.

Coping with the Busy Practice

When physicians with a 1,1 orientation find themselves in a busy practice, the difficulties encountered in trying to satisfy each patient outweigh the gain in income. As the patients stack up, the physician is likely to suggest that urgency is uncalled for and that the patients can get along just fine until the physician finds time to schedule surgery or perform an examination. Thus, the physician defers gathering information from the patient in the hope that this will somehow prevent the potentially worrisome responsibility of delivering medical care. The physician will agree to play the middleman, relaying requests for tests or treatment from the patient to the hospital or laboratory and back again, with no real concern as to whether or not the patient gets lost in the shuffle.

Even when surgery could be scheduled in a few days, if this is not the physician's norm, he or she is likely to say it cannot be done before the following week at the earliest. In this way the risk that something might misfire can at least be delayed. Spreading the patients out and decreasing the volume are the safest ways for the physician on a tightrope to avoid violation of the patients' expectations.

Scheduling and Time Management. "I don't need to schedule my activities. Patients contact me and their requests keep me busy enough."

The Hospital. "I keep up with what the hospital is doing, when I get time. The care delivered is really out of my hands once the patient reaches the ward. The patient talks to the nurse, the nurse talks to me, I talk to the patient, the patient talks to the nurse. You know how it goes."

Expenses. "I know how my expenses run. I keep them in line with everybody else's. Most people have too much office space, too many employees, and too new a carpet. I'm practical and I don't get any complaints."

Continuing Education. "I have learned more than most people learn in a lifetime. It's hands-on experience that pays off. These new studies can't even be read by most of us, and what they're proving this week will be disproved next week. I rely on common sense. It has always worked well for me."

Self-Evaluation. "I feel no need to review my performance. As long as patients are coming through that door, it tells me all I need to know."

Recognizing 1,1 Behavior

Many words can be used to describe 1,1-oriented behavior, but the phrases below depict in everyday language this style of medical leadership:

Appears unmotivated
Avoids genuine relationships
Defers and delays
Disclaims responsibility
Gives up easily
Has weak follow-through
Hopes to get by
Is likely to miss new things that need to be done

Is noncommittal
Is really just putting in time
Keeps out of the way
Lacks enthusiasm
Lets things run their course
Makes minimal effort
Volunteers few opinions
Waits for others to take action

Patient Reactions Based On Grid Styles

Patients want to be satisfied with medical care, and physicians can make a significant difference through the enthusiasm they display. Additionally, physicians can gain respect by showing patients how to follow through on treatments in order to get their fullest benefit. They can also help patients to see the unique application of a treatment to their particular situation and may even show patients why the treatment was the best use of their money. Unfortunately, the 1,1-oriented physician does none of these.

The 1,1 medical strategy is unlikely to be truly effective with any patients, whatever their Grid style. The only exception is when the treatment is clearly defined and no other physicians are around to better meet the patient need. Unless the patient already has a burning desire for the "right" treatment, which just happens to be offered by this physician, the 1,1 approach is unlikely to intrigue the patient at all.

9,1

When interviewing a 9,1-oriented patient, the 1,1-oriented physician inevitably meets resistance and confrontation. The physician's response is to withdraw immediately from any degree of commitment that may have already been made. This effectively prevents any combat between the patient and the physician. The patient's hostile statements have little effect on the physician's emotions, but they convey quite clearly the message that, "All bets are off." Mentally, the physician throws in the towel, saying, "What's the use. This patient is a real pain. I've got better things to do."

1,9

This physician is likely to misread the clues in the 1,9 patient's behavior. Rather than accurately interpreting the patient's desire for a relationship as the reason for an extended interview, the physician instead sees the patient as engaged in making a decision. Although this physician is impatient, the interview may continue until it becomes clear that the patient will not make a decision. The physician commonly sets up a future visit as a reasonable response to this indecision, the physician's hope being that the 1,9-oriented patient will not be so wishy-washy at their next meeting.

1,1

When the colorless and bland attitude of this physician is matched by that of patients equally as indifferent, an interesting relationship develops. Neither of these individuals has much use for the other. However, as the health of these patients has lapsed into a state that has prompted them to seek medical care, the physician can plug them into a diagnosis and provide treatment. If the treatment is routine and within the realm of the physician's expertise, the patient may receive appropriate care, even though the service is provided outside the realm of high-quality medical care and a genuine physician-patient relationship.

5,5

The uninterested and mechanical way in which a 1,1-oriented physician operates does little or nothing to meet the needs of a 5,5-oriented patient. This lack of involvement and enthusiasm does not inspire sufficient confidence to cause the patient to remain in treatment. A possible exception is when the physician's reputation, which was once prestigious, gets the attention of the patient. The 5,5-oriented patient is so status conscious that this may support a physician-patient relationship despite the physician. No possibility exists that the proposed therapy will be other than "tried and true," and this also appeals to this patient.

9,9

A physician operating in a 1,1 mode can anticipate unequivocal failure in dealing with a 9,9-oriented patient. Superficial knowledge will not impact a patient who is seeking sound solutions based on a thorough understanding of medical care. In some cases, the patient may draw the physician away from the 1,1 orientation by a confrontation that elevates the presentation to a more professional level. Even at that point, however, the lack of concern for the individual as a person is obvious and 9,9-oriented patients will move on, discouraged, but willing to put in the time to find physicians who can meet their medical and personal needs.

Summary

The physician with a 1,1 orientation has learned to be "out of it" while remaining in the practice of medicine. This physician gives no criticism and hopes to receive none. Though this is not a fairly common dominant style, it may occur when the physician is tired or burned out. Nonetheless, it is an unnatural approach to medical care. If this condition becomes chronic, the physician has probably slid progressively into this style in the face of defeat or overwhelming stress.

When a physician becomes discouraged by patients' attitudes toward him or her, this can create a never-ending cycle in which the 1,1 orientation leads the patient to be critical and the criticism is what perpetuates the 1,1 orientation.

What is the likely impact on success for a 1,1-oriented physician? The attitude is, "I accept the patients that come my way. This is my job, and I assume that my business will remain profitable." Because of the poor-quality outcomes that haunt this physician, he may in fact lose more money in lawsuits than is gained in a lifetime of practice. Patients will eventually decrease in number and, in a really competitive medical environment, this physician who once only constituted dead weight may become an unacceptably high financial risk to the hospital or insurance carrier that "provides his or her means for livelihood." Quality assurance programs are dedicated to finding and eliminating this style of medical care, even if it only occurs intermittently.

Chapter Eight

5,5 MEDICAL CARE: SEEKING THE SAFE PRACTICE

The doctors' lounge was filled with commotion and cigarette smoke. The smell of fresh coffee was the only thing that made the atmosphere bearable to John as he plowed through the mail, which had been crammed in the small cubicle with his physician number stenciled onto the door.

"Hey, John, how's it going? I noticed you're on the Peer Review Committee again this year. I was really glad to see that. We need more solid individuals like you who know how this hospital ought to work."

John smiled and sat down at the table of doctors.

"Hi, John. Listen, are you going to that utilization meeting tonight? You know, what's it called? There're so many of these HMOs and PPOs I can't keep them straight."

John sat up and smiled earnestly. "Oh, I'll be there. I belong to most of them and I think this meeting tonight is going to be really important. Somebody is going to bring up the issue of incorporating, so that we can act kind of like a union. I think these clowns have been walking on us long enough. Our fees have never been lower relative to the cost of living, and we've never had to see more patients just to keep up. I know we can't price-fix; that's illegal. But I think if we work within the system, we can apply enough pressure to get what we deserve. After all, we're only trying to get back to the status quo. It's not like we're out trying to gouge the public or something."

"You can say that again, John. Listen, are you staying pretty busy?"

John looked back with a big smile and said, "Sure, I couldn't be busier. If I could just get these third-party payers to deliver, I might be able to pay my bills!" The others laughed sympathetically.

"You know, John, I'd really like to see you as chairman of our department, to help get your sound thinking across to some of these people who just don't seem to care."

"Well, if I were chairman, I can tell you one thing; efficiency would get a damn sight more attention. If the hospitals could just save money, there wouldn't be so much peer review pressure on the physicians. I think the day of trying to order every lab test under the sun just to be sure we don't miss some obscure

diagnosis is over. Good medicine is efficient medicine.

"The patients are always going to want every little stone turned because that's what they've gotten used to, but I think it's our responsibility to make sure the system survives. After all, if the hospitals fail, we won't be able to deliver any medical care at all. You know, that's really all that PPOs and HMOs are trying to do — stay within the system and decrease the horrendous cost of medical care. I think if we just set up some solid rules and stick to them, patients are going to be fine and we won't have to suffer from all this unjustified criticism."

"Here, here, John, I think part of it's going to come down to peer review. We're going to have to start watching some of these turkeys who are ordering lab tests like they were interns on a medicine service."

"You're right. We've come to a point where no one needs to practice his own special brand of medicine. We know what the diagnoses are, and we see how the patients fit into them. I know everybody hates the word, but it's just a matter of making our own kind of cookbook and being sure that all the members of our organization stick to it. Those that don't are simply going to have to pay fines, or at least get public or peer exposure for wasting the system's money. After all, if we get to the end of the year and the money's gone, you know who has to come up with it."

John reached out and shook the hands of the three gentlemen who had supported all the things he had come to believe. These were trying times. Work had never been harder and remuneration never more complex. The paperwork required by the new organizations that came between him and the patient was almost overwhelming.

John passed by the nurses' station, just in time to answer the phone. The ward clerk, who had barely stood up, frowned as he took her seat.

"Hello. This is the private secretary of Susan Wilson speaking. May I help you?" Susan instantly changed her frown to a hearty laugh, and Dr. Smith handed her the phone.

"I know they'll eventually find a job description for me around here." He nudged her and winked, as they shared a laugh. Then he picked up his charts from the rack and began to make rounds on his patients.

"Hello, Jim. How's that leg?"

"Good to see you, John. It's doing just fine. Listen, they brought this form in here and told me I was supposed to sign it. I wasn't sure what it was all about — something about informed consent."

"Oh, yes, that's very important. You just need to sign that here, saying everything we did was okay with you.

"Well, I guess it's okay. I'm not really sure exactly what you did. I mean it's not like I had any reservations. After all..."

John interrupted, "Well, the clinic is certainly the best. And you know I wouldn't lead you astray."

"Yeah, that's for sure. Let me sign that thing. Do you need to witness it or anything?"

"No. It's really just a formality, but it's important that you fill it out so that we can put it on file."

As Jim scratched his name on the bottom line, he said, "Boy, I can hardly wait to get back to running. You know, I haven't been able to do anything very athletic for the last several years, but I'm sure looking forward to feeling like a kid again." He gave John a wink.

John smiled, realizing that the old boy was never going to feel quite like a kid, but reflecting his belief that showing a little enthusiasm about the future couldn't hurt anything. "You know, Jim, Dr. Nedderly was the first to describe the procedure we did on you, and I don't think anybody since has come up with a better way of doing it."

Jim looked reassured as John left the room.

Sue came running over and grabbed John's arm. "Dr. Smith, I almost forgot to tell you that Mr. Brown's family is really upset."

"Why? What happened?"

"Well, they claim you haven't been in to see the patient for two days."

Suddenly a blank expression came over John's face. He remembered old man Brown, angry and cantankerous from the first day he had come in the office. John had been forced to resort to every technique in the book to get Brown to consider surgery, even though it was clear that trying to improve the circulation was the best alternative to prevent amputation. Could it be possible that he hadn't seen the old man for two days?

"Well, Sue," John responded self-confidently, *"you know how families are. They're never here when you are in and out of the room, and if the patient is asleep, sometimes I don't interfere. I always check for problems by looking at your records and reviewing the resident's notes. After all, I haven't gotten a phone call, and if anything had gone wrong, you nurses would have let me know immediately."*

He smiled as if he had satisfied her concern and walked on into the patient's room. It wasn't the first time John had walked away from an angry patient, subconsciously putting distance between the patient and himself, hoping that a little time would help things cool off. This time he had gone a bit too far. Two days wasn't going to be overlooked.

"Hello, Mr. Brown. How are you doing, now that you've had time to really recover from our little surgery on your leg?"

Mr. Brown looked up, with one eye closed and the other one cocked, sort of demonstrating a perturbed acknowledgment that the physician had finally arrived. "Well, nice of you to drop by, doctor. Thought maybe you had kind of forgotten about me."

"No, no, Mr. Brown. Don't be silly. I've been extremely busy, and I've been called to emergencies several times when I've been on my way up here. But I've

kept tabs on you with the nurses, and they've reassured me that you've been doing just beautifully."

"Well, it's a good thing you weren't in here yesterday, or I'd have probably thrown you out the window. My leg hurts; it hurts bad. I don't think you've done me any good at all."

"Now, Mr. Brown. I never said that this operation was going to get you back on your feet. All we were trying to do was prevent an amputation."

"That's not the way I remember it. What good's a foot if you can't walk on it?"

"Now, Mr. Brown. You can look right here in the chart, and it says clearly that I explained all of the risks and benefits of this procedure to you.

"Yeah, yeah, sure, sure.

"Look, Mr. Brown. I know it's hard to see that now, but you made the right decision. You chose to be your best, to stand up for yourself and try to fight off this vascular disease. You should be proud of yourself."

The old man looked up, unconvinced and unimpressed.

"At any rate, you'll be home before you know it. The procedure we did is called the Elliott technique. It's been done thousands of times right here in the clinic, and it's gonna give you the best result possible. That's the bottom line. I think I'll let you out of here if you can calm your family down. I hear they're a little upset with me."

Mr. Brown looked out the window and said, "Yeah, they're upset with me too. The whole thing is pretty upsetting."

Choosing to ignore the innuendo, John replied, "I know how you feel, Mr. Brown. It's tough when the old body lets you down. But we'll do everything we can to make you better."

Dr. Smith turned and walked out of the room, ignoring the glare that Mr. Brown was giving him. He made a mental note that this would be their last encounter.

John arrived at his office on time, following his plan to see as many patients as possible while maintaining a smooth patient flow and keeping the accounts receivable stable. Corrine, his nurse, was skilled at rescheduling patients who were going to take more time than had been planned for in the schedule. The explanations were well memorized, and the patients were easy to deal with, as long as a lab test could be ordered that required review, records could be sent for, or any number of other excuses could be made to sound plausible.

The only rule Corrine had to follow was to be sure that patients were not unhappy and were not on their way to another physician as they went out the door.

Dr. Smith avoided extremes, never being the first to adopt a medical treatment nor the last to let one go. He had always considered his middle-of-the-road approach to medical practice ideal, until the fateful day when the subpoena for Mrs. Valerie Clark's medical record had come across his desk. He was sure *he had not done anything different with her, nothing out of the ordinary. Why would any patient sue him? He was in good standing, a member of all of the accepted professional organizations, and the most likely candidate to become chairman of his department this year. None of it was making much sense.*

As he thumbed through the brochures for continuing medical education and saw Tahiti and Barbados, he tried to decide which place would be more inviting at this time of year. He had been to countless conferences with countless experts and had always come away with virtually nothing new, and he felt tired, so why not have a little fun?

"I've done everything I'm supposed to," he reassured himself. "I've gotten all of my certificates of continuing medical education. I attend all of the hospital business meetings and grand rounds. I lecture the residents, give nursing in-services, practice exactly the way I'm supposed to. If doctors like me are getting sued, who's safe any more?"

General Characteristics of the 5,5-Orientation to Medicine

Less than a decade ago, most physicians would have found it unthinkable that the entire profession would be addressing the issue of what constitutes a "safe" practice. Throughout this chapter, the pressures that "new medicine," the PPOs, HMOs, DRGs, escalating malpractice insurance, and spiraling medical costs place on physicians to move toward the 5,5 style become apparent. The impact on quality may already be emerging.

The physician with a 5,5 perspective is in the middle, demonstrating an intermediate concern for production linked with a moderate concern for people. This physician is proud to be in the profession and is a steady performer who sets and reaches prescribed goals. However, such a person is not really striving to achieve excellence in medical performance or to create ideal relationships with patients. That, according to a 5,5-oriented physician, would be impractical. The justification is, "No matter how hard you try, you can only please some of the patients some of the time."

A successful 5,5 orientation reflects a physician striving for a sense of security and well-being. These good feelings may persist even when long-term quality issues are compromised for short-term convenience. The difficulty with the 5,5 style is that a contradiction between technical care and people's needs is presumed; that is, the 5,5 solution to the production/people, technical/human-need dilemma is to trade off, to give up half of one in order to get half of the other. The physician may even feel that people's needs are not completely realistic but that some effort is expected and must be exerted. The underlying assumption is that extreme positions promote conflict and should be avoided in favor of equilibrium. Steady progress comes from compromise, and the result is that a

5,5-oriented physician is unlikely to seek the best position for either quality medical care or the people involved.

Motivation

The primary underlying motivations of the 5,5-oriented physician are to belong, on the one hand, and to avoid embarrassment, almost at all costs, on the other. The positive motivation is to make progress within the system in order to belong and be a member in good standing. "I want to look good, to be 'in' with my colleagues." Being popular means exhibiting qualities that are respected in medical circles, including whatever is appropriate in dress, topics of conversation, the latest in medical-legal trivia, the "throw-away" journal article that everyone's talking about, and technical jargon related to the work itself. In order to be affable and companionable, this physician will be sociable, outgoing, and a good mixer, and, as a result, is likely to make many friends. A physician who is motivated to be "in" tends to keep relationships superficial and to take cues from the actions of others. Prevailing opinions become personal opinions. What others reject is rejected. The inclination is to embrace the traditions, precedents, and practices of medicine in a noncritical manner because "That's the best way" or "It's how things have always been done." The motivational motto is "If I think, look, and act like everyone else but a little more so, I will be a physician in good standing." The physician with a 5,5 orientation tends to identify with wealth and power, or with those who have it, and tries to gain prestige by association.

The negative motivation is to avoid being separated from the mainstream or becoming a target of ridicule. When this physician is unsuccessful and feels unpopular, out of step, and isolated from others, the experience may range from embarrassment to marked anxiety.

The 5,5-Oriented Physician-Patient Relationship

In order to identify the attributes of this physician style and what impact it will have on quality patient care as well as patient satisfaction, we will focus on the unique aspects of the 5,5 practice. This Grid style has special concerns and problems that need to be addressed as a means of understanding what constitutes excellent medical care in these times of rapid change.

Providing Patient Care

This physician has a straightforward philosophy about providing patient care: avoid malpractice, maintain an adequate income, enjoy the prestige of being a physician, and keep from being singled out or faulted by medical peers. The underlying motive is to deliver the medical care that the system is capable of producing within the rules.

Communication. The 5,5 communication leaves the physician feeling self-confident and ready to handle any patient who has come for conventional medical care. However, the interview follows a standard format, well rehearsed and well supported by precedents or past practices. The difficulty comes in individualizing care and recognizing needs that do not fit the categories this physician has learned to depend on.

5,5-oriented physician has a preset agenda of questions worked out and has arranged to move patients indirectly toward the physician's point of view. The strategy is fixed, yet the tactics are flexible. Thus, the second, third, and fourth questions are calculated to engage the patient's interest and to promote involvement. The second question asked is a function of the answer to the first. The third question is being mentally rehearsed while the physician displays great interest in the information being given in answer to the second question, and so on. However, this "prepackaged" quality quickly becomes apparent to anyone who recognizes that the questions are intended to maneuver the patient in a planned direction. As a result, patients are unlikely to be aroused to either real participation or resistance by this type of pseudosophisticated, shallow interrogation. By the end of the interview, the patient will have been introduced to and agreed with all facets of the proposed treatment.

Establishing patient expectations. A 5,5-oriented physician respects the truth but exercises flexibility in seeking and interpreting what the truth is. While what is said is correct, what is left unsaid or what is implied may allow conclusions to be drawn that are not fully justified. When confronted with the dilemma of making an invalid statement as opposed to remaining silent, this physician is very conscious of "how things look on the record," "what is in the chart," and "never saying things that can't be backed up" — all 5,5 concerns. Whatever the "sins" are, they are all sins of omission. This legalistic concept of integrity ensures that the statements made are true, yet may allow misunderstandings that will lead the patient to believe that the treatment is more useful than it really is. When the patient ultimately becomes disillusioned, the physician accepts no responsibility for the misconceptions, referring to the statements that were carefully documented in the course of care.

Bluffing is another way to shade the truth. This occurs when the physician becomes committed to doing something in the hope of a good outcome, even in the face of realistic doubts about the possibility of achieving it. This kind of a bluff is also found in the 9,1 orientation, with the difference that the 9,1-oriented physician "moves hell and high water" to make things happen and in this way may avoid being held accountable. By comparison, the 5,5 attitude is to have a bundle of excuses ready in case the hope is not realized and he or she is confronted.

The patient's reaction to 5,5-oriented physician bluffing tactics, once aware of them, is likely to be "You have to take everything this physician says with a grain of salt." The patient soon learns to discount the actual words and to read between the lines. Expectations for quality are low because trust has been compromised.

Acquiring Knowledge. This physician knows something about everything but is not an expert on anything. Information sources, such as medical journals, are likely to get attention only as a buffer to the physician's being held accountable or to score a one-upmanship point. Otherwise, they are given a cursory review. One of the ways a 5,5-oriented physician rationalizes this superficial approach is to say, "Ask me the question you want answered, and I'll get the information you desire."

The physician stays informed, at least in general terms, about the organizational changes of the hospital, the trends being established by other physicians, and what the competition is. The physician keeps track of new patients who had been seeing other physicians. Derogatory remarks are usually avoided as they might have to be defended at a later time. Acknowledging other physicians with faint praise tells the patient that the past provider was honest, but it also avoids giving competitors a boost. Once enough information has been gathered about past care to fit the patient comfortably into a "diagnosis," discussion about previous care is dropped.

If this physician is a member of organization delivering medical care, the typical approach to gathering knowledge will use actuarial review to clarify the accepted methods for creating a safe, profitable approach to medical care. To stay "in" with the other members of the organization, the physician is likely to have built up a repertoire of up-to-date knowledge on sports and information about local happenings, as well as political stories that are making the rounds. All of this is invaluable for establishing and maintaining friendly contacts with peers and patients.

To sum up, the physician's knowledge, whether of therapy, patients, or peers, tends to be shallow. The objective of acquiring such knowledge is to create rapport or to shield the physician from exposure to criticism by the patient, peer review committee, lawyers, and, in some cases, the employer-administrator.

Assessing the patient's needs. The basic 5,5 assumption is that the patient's felt needs or expressed needs are the ultimate point of departure for a needs analysis. The goal is to appeal to the patient, so finding out what the patient feels or thinks is paramount. Being alert to clues in what the patient is saying may identify particular tendencies, interests, or emotions to which the physician can appeal. Even if the physician realizes that the felt need is not the real need, challenging the prospect is resisted, as that is more work than is necessary. The result is that the physician attempts to match a treatment to what the patient wants, even though assisting the patient in diagnosing the real problem might lead to a better decision. The treatment, taken from a "cafeteria line" of therapies, is likely to be remarkably similar to that of other physicians working under similar pricing schemes, and the price tends to be "what the market will bear."

Every experienced physician has had a patient whose expressed needs were not the best reflection of actual needs. When the contract for care rests on decisions based on felt needs rather than real medical needs, patients are likely to become dissatisfied if they realize that the quality of the outcome was not what they were really after. The problem goes back to the 5,5 style of listening, which pigeonholes each remark according to some preestablished system of interpretation. The major difficulty is that no frame of reference can be so refined as to catalog all the nuances of thought and feelings that characterize the presentations of patients. Each is unique; all are different. Thus, the 5,5-oriented physician's restricted scope of listening is likely to lead to answers that, while they may appear relevant, are not completely on target. With time, these restricted categories of care come to represent the only answers this physician knows how to give, and the result is a far cry from high quality, let alone medical excellence.

Decision Making. The 5,5-oriented physician has little difficulty in making quick decisions based on precedent. However, decision making becomes difficult when the decision being considered might be unpopular, be unpleasant, or lead to new and untested situations.

Delegation is the answer. Although done in the name of equity and fairness, it really means that responsibilities or problems are carved up, with "everybody" given a fair share. This may be sound when the solution to a problem is purely mechanical, but the solutions for many medical problems call for different contributions based on different abilities.

Another problem is that popularity rather than objective evidence is used to decide what is right or valid. This means that several people may agree on the same assumptions, even when they are faulty. The greater the popularity, the greater the risk of accepting such majority agreements as being based on objective facts, even when they are not. "Group thinking" is a special case of a 5,5 orientation. Unsure of themselves or their facts, such individuals prefer to go along and to give their support rather than to engage in thorough inquiry, advocate for their real convictions, or create opposition to an emerging plan. Under this kind of decision making, the plan snowballs and rolls over what few reservations may remain. No one wants to be out of step. So agreement is reached, an action is taken, and a medical fiasco results. At the fullest development of this scenario, a vital piece of information may be overlooked to avoid criticism. The physician may look away when others use questionable methods, stating, "Everybody does it." The ability to shift, twist, turn, and yet stay with the majority guides all decisions made under the 5,5-oriented physician style until integrity falls by the wayside.

Bending the truth, half-truths, or white lies may become acceptable tactics for reaching a decision. Over a period of time, such distortions are likely to form a patchwork of contradictions, which then require even more squirming. The philosophy that evolves is that "the end justifies the means" as long as no one is caught. This is not conscious manipulation of the sort associated with a facade (Appendix B) or premeditated lying. A 5,5-oriented physician is not likely to realize how the tailoring of information in order to persuade others may color his or her understanding.

Advocacy in the area of decision making is not determined by convictions but by what is politically safe and workable. This can have important implications for medical ethics. A 5,5-oriented physician may operate under no particular ethical compulsion beyond "doing what everybody else is doing." This can result in an erosion of medical ethics and morality until they become purely situational. A foundation of equity and justice may actually be lost if no one is prepared to question prevailing attitudes that are ethically unsound.

Level of responsibility. The 5,5-oriented physician unknowingly accepts full responsibility for an outcome by using several clever but tricky techniques to give the patient the illusion of participation. One way is to convert declarative statements into questions with which the patient can be expected to agree:

Physician: Isn't this equipment impressive?
Patient: Yes, it looks really complicated.
Physician: Looks like it ought to do the job, don't you think?
Patient: Yes, it certainly does.

Figuratively, hand-in-hand down a path strewn with "yes blossoms," the physician leads the patient to a final acceptance of therapy. The proposition is made quite undramatically. It becomes just a matter of routine to answer "yes." If patients do not understand why they came to agree with treatment, their tendency is to give full responsibility for the quality of the outcome to the physician.

Another variant of pseudoparticipation through questioning is the "cathedral chimes" technique. Again, the intention is to get the patient habituated to making a positive reply. This time, however, the emphasis is on the personal reward of making the right decision. With health maintenance and preferred provider organizations, these physicians may find themselves involved in conversations like the following. Note the harmonious chiming effect of the declarative statements posed as questions: "Mr. Brown, you do understand our plan is going to save you money?" (The unverbalized answer, but the one the patient is expected to feel, is, "Yes, of course I do.) "I'm sure you feel your family would greatly benefit through insuring good health?" ("Oh, yes, I do.") "And surely you appreciate the freedom from worry that this would give you and your family?" ("Yes, yes.") By now the patient's original reason for seeking care is secondary to the overwhelmingly clear decision to go with the plan and to continue getting excellent care for the entire family.

As for the patient's felt needs, when they cannot be matched because of the unavailability of therapy or the price, the 5,5-oriented physician attempts to bring the patient to an intermediate position. This is the most accepted basis for a decision in the buy-sell relationship today. Pseudoparticipation and involvement quite often are dominated by attempts to reach solutions on therapy, cost, discounts, and so on by accommodating differences. The responsibility of the patient is that of a buyer and the biggest problem that can arise in any buy-sell relationship is that the customer will want a refund if the quality of the product falls short of expectations.

Initiative. The status quo defines the arena of action for this physician. The objective is to run operations in an orderly manner. The exercise of initiative is limited; novel or experimental approaches are seen as untried and risky. Creative ideas often lead to remarks such as, "Better not," "A word of caution...," "A little too radical...," or "I wish it were that easy...." The 5,5-oriented physician only feels free to act if precedents are already established. He or she is more likely to ask, "Do they do it that way at the university?" or, if highly conscious of prestige, at an institution recognized as a leader in the particular specialty. Unless pressured otherwise, he or she will continue to say, "Too risky."

When opinions, policies, and regulations are ambiguous, or when more than one majority opinion exists, the 5,5-oriented physician turns to a consultant for guidance. In this way the physician is seen as initiating and exercising responsibility.

Conflict Resolution. The 5,5 approach is based on an internal logic that says, "No person or treatment philosophy has ever been completely right. Therefore, skill is needed to adjust to the inevitable conflicts that occur in daily medical management."

Preventing conflict. Conflict related to independent judgment is avoided by carefully adhering to established protocols and thereby feeling safe and secure. A 5,5-oriented physician often venerates traditions and long-established practices.

As long as performance conforms to them, everything is regarded as moving in an appropriate manner, and conflicts are unlikely to arise.

Falling back on diplomacy is another method used to prevent conflict. Diplomatic skills allow relationships to be structured according to preset conventions that honor status, hierarchy, and seniority. Achieving status within the hierarchy may result in the sacrifice of self-expression and spontaneity, but this physician is willing to pay that price.

Making rules, bylaws, standards, or policies or emphasizing existing ones reduces the likelihood of person-to-person conflict. Rules can be produced to cover everything; but we are rapidly learning that, once made, rules tend to take on a life of their own. When relied on as a substitute for direct communication, they can stifle initiative and be seen as a trap by those involved.

Because taking a stand can put one physician at odds with others, the 5,5 approach is to discover in advance whether disagreements with a position are likely to be encountered. If a position will spark disagreement, it can be modified or abandoned. The key is to remain unlinked to controversial positions.

Handling conflict when it appears. This physician feels that it is unwise to confront conflict directly, because when a disagreement becomes polarized someone wins and someone loses. The loser then becomes a potential enemy. So, when possible, the physician attempts to back off and let tensions in the situation cool.

The 5,5 approach is often to take some part of everyone's idea and come up with a halfway solution. It may not be perfect, but it is often accepted. The physician's goal is to find a middle position in preference to continuing to fight. However, this may not meet the full requirements of anyone, and it can leave reservations and doubts in the mind of the patient.

The best care is rarely defined by something that represents a splitting of differences between divergent points of view. Therein lies the problem.

When conflict remains. This physician may react to conflicts that persist in several ways, and although any of them may calm the situation on the surface, the disagreements usually remain.

Accepting impasse. A 5,5 practice for living with disagreement in organizational structures such as the hospital is expressed in the idea, "We agree to disagree." Because skills of conflict solving do not exist, areas of disagreement are avoided rather than trying to find the reasons and relieve them. This approach applied to patients can be a disaster. What serves as a rationalization for inaction in the bureaucracy of hospitals and other organizations delivering medical care is likely to create anger on the part of patients who are not willing to have their disagreements ignored.

Distancing. When conflict remains unsolved, this physician hopes that tensions will dissipate before seeing the patient again or by discussing only topics that do not provoke disagreement. This attempt to sidestep is actually a withdrawal from the real issue.

All of these techniques of conflict resolution fall short because of their dependency on a compromise philosophy. At the point of disagreement, the patient demands more than half attention, and with the rapidly advancing technology of medicine, holding on to the status quo too long can result in a physician slipping accidentally outside the standards of care. Beyond these limitations, the physician misses an opportunity to grow and change, as self-evaluation is a forgotten benefit of sound conflict resolution.

Dealing with patient objections. Physicians who are 5,5 oriented take care to avoid getting out on an emotional limb that anybody could cut off. This conservative approach shelters such people from risk, but it can also deprive them of the richness of living. It makes these physicians seem mechanical and emotionally shallow. To "fit the situation," they respond as expected rather than according to true feelings.

The 5,5 way of treating interruptions is a good example. This physician appreciates that patients are often disposed to talk about matters not directly relevant to the patient-physician interview. These interruptions are seen not as objections but rather as detours on the road to acceptance. The interruption is acknowledged by a courteous pause. The physician listens to whatever is said and tries to connect it with a preestablished part of the interview. If no connection is evident, the physician nevertheless hears the patient out, making some bland remark such as, "That's very interesting," and then shifts back to the main route. Emotions are not part of the process.

Rather than dealing with objections according to the patient's unique frame of reference, the physician may seek to introduce benefits that counteract the stated objection. Then, it is hoped, the patient will say something like, "Well, I guess my objection is really not very important in light of the total situation you have presented."

The 5,5-oriented physician believes that a perfect fit between what can be done and what the patient wants done is a rarity indeed. Therefore, he or she may yield to the patient's objection and modify the patient's care accordingly. After all, there are many ways of making an approximation almost a perfect fit, and the patient's objection may be partially justified due to the current limitations of medicine.

Finally, because of a high reliance on the tried-and-true presentation, this physician is particularly vulnerable when vigorously probed by the patient. When this 5,5 technique is punctured, the physician is likely to be unable to cope, because prepared responses do not exist for a unique situation.

Critique and Feedback. The 5,5 approach to critique and feedback is based on the notion of positive reinforcement — by complimenting coworkers and patients on their good performance and by receiving compliments in return. Negative feedback is risky because it can backfire. This physician wants happy patients and popularity with peers and coworkers, even though he or she realizes the importance of being aware of weaknesses in order to improve. One way of dealing with negative information is indirectly, by asking patients a question that, if answered objectively, forces the patients to acknowledge their weaknesses. If that does not work, the topic is likely to be dropped. Another way to make a negative or critical reaction more acceptable is to sandwich a criticism in between two compliments. This makes it easier for the patient to accept. It also may cloud the issue that better compliance is needed to effect a cure.

This approach to giving patients feedback is not candid or straightforward. The result is misunderstanding, because the message is not likely to be clear. This deficiency in the style of feedback is hard to recognize and harder to correct, because this physician has become so familiar with the statement, "They didn't comply with my instructions; there wasn't anything I could do about it." The question of why they did not comply is not asked; rather their behavior is assumed to be "typical of patients these days."

Informed consent. Informed consent is viewed as a hospital regulation, a series of statements mechanically logged into a chart according to the rules that protect the hospital and physician, thus ensuring the safe practice. Because the physician's aim is solely to bring about agreement on the part of the patient, true understanding of the information delivered is immaterial.

A variety of techniques are utilized to influence this outcome, including the silent treatment, seed planting, and the use of rhetorical questions that elicit the answer the physician wants from the patient, along with a multitude of other sales techniques. The result is undoubtedly the signing of an informed consent contract, but because true understanding is assumed to be an impossibility, winning the patient over replaces the education that lets the patient participate in the decisions about medical care.

If the contract is signed, the 5,5-oriented physician is eager to compliment the patient on an excellent decision, the soundness of reaching it, and the deep satisfaction that will be derived from having exercised such solid decision making. This unadulterated use of positive reinforcement coincides with the need many people experience to be accepted by others as reasonable and thoughtful people who have exercised good judgment. A critical difference is that the physician's reinforcement strategies constitute a selling technique rather than an effort to genuinely involve the patient in decision making toward the best medical care. The patient, having left the office and having begun to reflect on the decision, even though satisfied with it, is likely to develop a sense of uneasiness. The patient may even become distrustful of the physician's integrity, wary about being engulfed in further encounters. Because the patient has been controlled, no real responsibility for the decision is felt, and that is a dangerous medical-legal situation if a perfect outcome does not result.

New and Established Patients

The attitude underlying a 5,5 orientation is that the gateway to a patient's mind surely opens when the patient can be engaged in conversation that presents the physician as an attractive personality. A professional air, coupled with a friendly approach, is conveyed.

Physician: Hi. I'm Dr. John Smith. You can call me Jack if you like.
Patient: It's nice to meet you, Dr...., er, Jack. My name is Elizabeth Green.
Physician: Liz for short, right?
Patient: Uh, yes.
Physician: I'm happy to meet you. I see that Jackie Newton gave you our name. It's nice to have the opportunity to help you out.
Patient: How exactly does your clinic work?
Physician: I'm glad you asked. It's important for you to know you're in the right place. Ha! Ha! We are the oldest clinic west of the Mississippi. We've been at it steadily for 30 years now. So you can see our record speaks for itself. We know how to make things work. Now what brought you in?

The opening phase may include a review of mutual acquaintances or a brief discussion of general interest topics, all designed to help the patient move into an easy give-and-take conversation and feel accepted as an intelligent, alert person.

Having approximately the same concern for people as for the therapy, being reasonably well informed on many subjects, and taking the patient's tempo, the 5,5-oriented physician gains a reputation for being an easy person with whom to discuss medicine. The character of the discussion shifts in a subtle way, however. In the beginning, the physician listens to pick up the patient's interests and attitudes; near the end of the interview, the direction shifts to focusing on the major themes, attitudes, and feelings that will ensure that a patient is satisfied with therapy.

If a favorable climate is not established through this technique, or if the patient appears uninterested, the physician moves quickly into another technique that is geared to produce patient participation, whether genuine or not. As an example, if the patient shows suspicion or doubt about surgery as the only option for care, the 5,5-oriented physician will go back to comments about the social strain of the illness or the pressure that will be placed on the family. The inference made is that the choice is an either-or one: Take the treatment or suffer more family and social difficulties. The bottom line for this physician is to keep the patient coming back.

The 5,5-oriented physician actively nurtures established patients, without pressing too hard. Beyond the value of keeping in touch for maintaining patient-physician relationships, casual friendships that permit the exchange of information, rumors, and so on are in themselves quite satisfying. When appropriate, advantage is taken of club memberships, luncheons, afternoon golf, tennis matches, or a drink in the club room in order to cement a patient relationship or a peer referral.

Another way of maintaining patients is through scheduling regular visits to respond to any difficulty that may have developed. A goal is to focus the patient's attention on something new and different during each successive visit. Even though some of the new medical facts are trivial, this physician emphasizes their importance in order to maintain interest. Advice may have no direct connection to ongoing care but may involve a tidbit of information, a suggestion about a vacation, a new way of thinking about social situations, or any interesting health trend that the physician may have learned from another patient in a similar conversation. These social interactions in the office are more than "touching base." They are used to seek further referrals from those patients, who come to enjoy the physician's latest medical news story and tips on improving health.

Coping with the Busy Practice

The 5,5-oriented physician is more than pleased to be busy. If the patient volume increases to a point of overload, the approach to the problem is to move patients toward an "equilibrium" level. Patients will continue to receive treatment but, at times, in smaller doses. An example is the patient who obviously needs surgery but is rescheduled to a day that is less busy, with the explanation that lab tests must be drawn and then a reconsideration of therapy may be necessary. The actual intention is to keep patients in the system and, through this kind of compromise, the patient's needs are at least partially met. No one is entirely satisfied, but no one is left completely frustrated. More importantly, the risk of exposing this patient to another physician as possible competition is reduced, though of course not entirely eliminated.

Scheduling and Time Management. "I make my plans according to what I know my patients will accept and what I know they will resist. After explaining my goals for therapy and the time schedules that must be met, I double-check to make sure my patients agree with my plans. It really can work out quite nicely for everyone involved."

The Hospital. "I like people who fit in. I touch bases informally to discuss how things are going. I tend to emphasize good points and avoid appearing critical or negative. My coworkers at the hospital know that I take their thoughts and feelings into account in my decisions."

Expenses. "I usually keep my expenses within standard guidelines. At times, additional expenditures may help me create a better market. That's the way the game is being played these days."

Continuing Education. "I keep up with my continuing medical education requirements and attend the hospital-sponsored grand rounds and business meetings. I think this kind of support for continuing medical education is critical and helps everybody reach an acceptable level of performance. It's important to know how others are doing things in this day and age, when you are punished legally for doing anything different."

Self-Evaluation. "I take frequent hard looks at myself to identify where I may be out of step. I try to take a positive approach with myself and others. Positive suggestions motivate, but criticism turns people off, myself included."

Recognizing 5,5 Behavior

The following words and phrases give the flavor of the 5,5-oriented physician as described in daily activities:

Accommodates
Cautious
Compromises
Conformist
Evasive when challenged
Expedient
Indirect
Likes the tried and true
Negotiates
Prefers middle ground
Prefers to act on precedent
Pulls punches
Sandwiches bad between good comments
Soft-pedals disagreement
Stays on the majority side
Straddles issues
Swallows convictions in the interest of progress

Tests the wind
Waffles
Waits to see where others stand

Patient Reactions Based On Grid Styles

Because the 5,5-oriented physician is controlled by patient's actions and reactions, regardless of Grid style, the interview is usually paced in accord with the patient's mood, moving rapidly along when the patient is enthusiastic and slacking off when the patient shows doubt. The patient becomes the physician's metronome. This physician's finely tuned ability to use "sales techniques," coupled with a personal approach to integrity that permits certain details to be left out that might be disadvantageous to reaching agreement, oftentimes causes a patient to make commitments without full awareness of the facts or, for that matter, without even realizing that a commitment has been made.

Patients' reactions to 5,5 medical care vary. The physician's strategy is likely to succeed with patients who are in a hurry or whose fears prevent them from concentrating fully on the criteria for making a sound decision. Almost all patients can be swayed by subtle suggestions at one time or another. However, all the patient has to do is to detect a false note in the physician's instructions and certain suspicions are aroused. Watching and listening ever more closely, the patient may begin to see through the surface film of illusion.

9,1

To a 9,1-oriented patient, a 5,5 medical approach has a hollow ring and is unconvincing. The physician's knowledge is too superficial to give this patient confidence. Objections are parried and deflected rather than being handled with factual answers expressed with the conviction that wins approval.

In order to "fight," a 9,1-oriented patient needs something to push against. This physician is so flexible that a shift in position can be made on a moment's notice. This defense mechanism allows the physician to avoid polarizing issues, but a patient who feels trapped or victimized by the physician's technique may take an aggressive stance. The 5,5-oriented physician's inclination is to continue with a tried-and-true routine, attempting to stay on the predetermined track and to overcome interruptions and objections when they occur. The physician tries to forestall future objections by expanding the information to answer possible questions in advance. This continues to the point when the patient expresses dislike for the suggested care, becomes impatient and openly hostile, and finally terminates the interview, saying, "Let me think about it," or, simply, "No way."

The physician's moderate energy and enthusiasm, and the gimmicks that characterize the 5,5 technique are not likely to move 9,1-oriented patients out of the 9,1 Grid style. The physician does not level with patients in a way that encourages shared responsibility, and if treatment ensues, these angry patients will demand that the physician prove their suspicions and doubts were unwarranted by giving them perfect outcomes.

1,9

The 5,5 approach is more likely to be successful with a 1,9-oriented patient because this patient's goal is to please and not to arouse anxiety. The presentation is exciting to a patient who wants to be liked and is thus motivated to say, "yes." Although the physician may not fully satisfy the patient's desire for a warm personal relationship, the patient will probably move positively toward the desired agreement on issues of treatment. Difficulties for this physician begin when the time for informed consent arrives. Although the patient has indicated "yes" all along, there may now be an unwillingness to proceed. Rather than saying "no," the patient simply tries to defer the decision. In this way, the 1,9-oriented patient avoids being blatantly negative but still avoids a "yes" decision. If the physician presses forward at this point instead of accepting excuses, the patient will probably make the decision to accept treatment. However, if expectations are not fulfilled later on, the patient feels let down, hurt, and disappointed. Trust is eroded, high quality is in no way assured, and a high medical-legal risk may have been created.

1,1

The physician is quick to recognize the key difference between patients with a 1,9 and a 1,1 orientation. Whereas the 1,9-oriented patient responds affirmatively to the programmed questions of a 5,5 presentation, the 1,1-oriented patient responds with grunts or well-aimed silence. Rather than taking this silence as an indication of "zero interest" and becoming discouraged, the 5,5-oriented physician continues to "sell" information, closely following a number of well-rehearsed techniques. This patient is easy to deal with because both physician and patient respond to the same kind of signals. The patient's lack of interest concerning in-depth medical knowledge fits the physician's superficial level of research. Because the patient's desires are formulated in conventional terms and are met by tried-and-true therapy, the patient finds nothing abrasive in this approach. The physician responds to the style of this patient and moves at a tempo harmonious enough to ensure that treatment will be delivered.

5,5

The 5,5 approach is most natural and successful with a 5,5-oriented patient.

Because this patient comes into the medical situation with a prestige-centered orientation and the physician is tuned to respond to this need, the two individuals often work well together and really "hit it off." The proposed treatment fits the patient's preconceptions, and agreement about care is likely to come easily.

9,9

The 9,9-oriented patient finds this physician unconvincing, unless the therapy or advice just happens to solve a real need. Usually, the patient wants more facts about the treatment, more logical explanation to support the physician's claims for the merits of the approach, and more information about the therapy's risks and benefits as they relate to the patient's needs. Generally the 5,5-oriented physician is unable to provide this detailed information.

As the physician-patient interaction unfolds, the patient makes the effort to uncover the physician's true depth of knowledge and commitment to meeting the patient's needs. Upon being subjected to this patient's problem-solving approach, the physician may demonstrate either a high level of competence or virtual incompetence. The physician operating under 5,5 assumptions finds it difficult to deal successfully with a 9,9-oriented patient, even though the opportunity for a successful outcome is quite good, particularly if the physician takes the patient's lead and gathers the relevant facts and information required for an insight-based decision. 9,9-oriented patients bring enthusiasm and commitment to their care. This way of participating in the interview and the nature of their questions invite more openness and candor on the physician's part and greater clarity in specifying what the therapy can and cannot do. The physician who responds to the patient's initiatives shifts from a 5,5 dominant style into a 9,9 back-up. If the shift is not made, the patient will go elsewhere.

Summary

The 5,5-oriented physician is not charged with high energy, and the physician-patient interview does not genuinely involve the patient. The conviction and commitment it evokes may be strong enough to produce agreement at the time, but, being somewhat illusory, the basis for agreement tends to vanish afterward. The 5,5 approach is often effective, however, particularly when a patient desires personal association with a prestigious practice or when a clear need exists for a highly reputable therapy.

A 5,5-oriented physician wants to build prestige and to avoid being labeled as odd or different. Being seen as a good doctor in the eyes of patients, coworkers, and peers is important. By respecting traditions, supporting the status quo, and avoiding behavior that might be viewed as deviating from the norm, this physician gains the kind of reputation that provides a career path to security.

Using insurance price structures closely as a guide, a 5,5-oriented physician can be expected to put the same degree of emphasis on profit as does the physician community. The attitude is, "Reasonable profit is built into our price structure and is necessary to keep the office running."

This physician feels that it is impossible to realize a profit without taking new patients, at a lower profit margin, such as that offered in managed care contracts with HMOs, PPOs, or hospitals. This attempt to "stay busy" leads to an increased load and an even greater temptation to maintain the controls that epitomize a 5,5-oriented practice. Profit levels may increase, but the important issue is that they at least be stabilized so that this physician sees the means for survival in a rapidly changing medical community. These moves are justified because only a slight degree of "drag" is introduced into the system and "Everybody else is doing it." The physician works to keep his or her share of established accounts and to replace lost accounts with new business, even if it means additional hours and a reduction in the quality of life — all the while complaining that the system has changed, third-party payers and increased overhead are to blame, and work has never been harder.

The quality result of this type of care is what the system has set as the rule. To achieve care that is above the 5,5 standard is called outstanding and to fall below this standard is difficult to defend in court. The danger of making this style of care your goal is that under stress it is a short fall to the 1,1 corner and the compromises in quality care that await you there.

Chapter Nine

9,9 MEDICAL CARE: INTEGRATING THE QUALITIES OF EXCELLENCE

Dr. Tom Jones leaned back on the couch and stretched his back. Everybody else was still sitting cross-legged on the floor finishing dinner. "Boy, that was good, Paul. Did you really cook all of this?"

Paul looked up with a big smile.

Dr. Jones continued, "You know it's hard to believe, but I'd give up medicine if I could cook like that! Maggie, I'm moving in; one more rib and I'll be in heaven."

Paul, in his usual slow drawl, said, "It's nothing really. If I'd had a few more hours, I could've gotten them tender." Paul smiled in the irresistible way that endeared him to most people on first meeting.

"That's what I like. The best ribs I've ever had, and he's not even happy with them." Laughter filled the room, and the sense of camaraderie permeated the atmosphere.

Kevin interjected, "Say, Tom, I'd heard you are a doctor. Are times really that tough? My boy is in practice in Oregon, and he says between competition, malpractice, and something called capitation, that he can hardly pay his bills. He says he can't quit because an insurance 'tail' would cost him thousands of dollars even after he'd stopped seeing patients. And he keeps talking about 'high-risk patients,' whatever that means."

Tom looked deeply at the elderly gentleman to see if he was genuinely interested in a reply. "Well, high risk; he probably means that these days sick patients are more likely to bring a lawsuit if they get a bad outcome. All patients are a little risky to take care of these days." The room became quiet. Tom could tell that this wasn't going to be one of those parties where everyone asked him for free medical advice.

Kevin started it off. "You know, it makes me sick to see all the time that boy put into school and to hear him moan about trying to make as good a salary as

I had already been making for 10 years when I was his age."

"Oh, I think doctors do all right. Mine still manages to drive a BMW or Mercedes, maybe it's a Rolls Royce. I can't get too concerned." Maggie frowned. Tom could tell some experience had turned her sour.

Just then Wendell spoke up, "Well, present company excluded, I think it's hard to find a good doctor. I mean, I got a nail in my foot and went to one of those Doc-in-a-Box places. The doctor told me to keep it dry and said if it was too deep I might need a specialist. He didn't give me any antibiotics, just said if it got worse to call. Well, I didn't go there to find out what to do if it got worse.

"So then I was telling my friend Dr. Noble about why I was missing our golf match, and his first questions were, 'What are you soaking it in?' and 'What antibiotics are you on?' Well, I told him I was wrapping it in cellophane when I took a shower, and he broke out laughing. Then he went to the store, got me some solution to soak it in, and gave me antibiotics. And now look. I can stand on it, no pain, nothing. I mean, that's a real doctor; he has a little common sense. That Doc-in-a-Box would have had me back in sick as a dog. By now I probably would have been shuffled to a specialist for some kind of surgery."

Karen was rising to the discussion. She barked, "And the specialist would probably have given you the wrong drug."

"Yeah," Maggie chimed in, "I'd much rather go to a family doctor, someone who knows the whole family. If he can't take care of it, he gets someone who can. My GP is our friend, and I just love him."

Tom smiled, "Sounds like he has established a good rapport." Everyone laughed a bit uneasily. "I mean, the system is getting really complex. Americans expect the best possible care. They want specialty skills but they don't want to lose the feeling of rapport that a family doctor provides. This doctor is supposed to take care of the entire family but also know when to get the patient to the right specialist."

Looking directly at Karen, "For some, I don't think any specialist is going to be good enough. You know, the wrong drug." Tom smiled sincerely.

Karen sat up, and it was easy to see by the look in her eye that the war was on. "I got more help from a chiropractor than I ever got from any specialist, and when I have my baby, I'm going to deliver at home by a midwife — someone who only has four patients at a time and can be reached day or night."

Maggie spoke up, looking out over her pregnant abdomen. "What will you do if you get into an emergency?" She felt the baby kick. "I'm going to be in a hospital!"

Tom leaned forward. "I know what you're talking about, Maggie. I have covered midwives before, but the key word is covered. *Time is the critical factor. I gave it up because I couldn't accept the difficulty of coming in from home to meet someone I didn't know who was in a life-and-death situation. Patients who don't know any more about you than that you are the specialist expect you to come in and save the day." Tom was maintaining a comfortable poise, giving personal experience and not attacking in any way. "You said yourself, or at least what I heard, is that you don't trust specialists. That's not too good for me, the specialist."*

Karen glared back, "Well I've got reason. Just read the papers."

"I know." Dr. Jones leaned back, feeling the battle ready to come to resolution. "I spend a lot of time thinking about the things you've said, Karen. You are not alone. As a matter of fact, I've been studying some of these problems, and a lot of it boils down to communication."

Karen looked skeptical. She was listening for the usual doctor-protecting-doctor defense she had come to expect from her long history of grilling physicians at occasions such as this one.

Tom went on. "People use six main styles of communication to relate to each other." Tom stopped and chuckled. "Now, you are using what I call a 9,1 orientation, Karen."

Karen jumped out of her chair. "Whoa, a 9,1. I'm not even a person now. I've been reduced to a number."

Tom looked down and smiled as the room filled with laughter. "I really hadn't planned a lecture, but let me see if I can get out of this one. What do you look for in a doctor?"

The room was quiet. Karen was still glaring.

Wendell broke the silence. "Gotta be good." Maggie added, "But, caring."

"That's right, equal amounts of both. What we call 9,9, which is really just being a 9 on a scale of 1 to 10. You know there are no real 10s."

Tension was easing, and smiles began to fill the room.

"Now a 9,1-oriented doctor is the one you've been describing, Karen — good, but he crams it down your throat. You're not a person, just a medical problem, and a challenge to his medical knowledge."

Karen was still preparing herself for battle, as she moved to the edge of her chair.

"Now, we've all agreed that the 9,9 orientation for doctors is ideal, but let's look at it the other way around. Who gets the best care in medicine? Not surprisingly, the patient with the same qualities, one who is concerned about getting well and is probably well-read like you, Karen. But added to this is something surprising. The 9,9-oriented patient, the one who gets the best care, cares about the physician as a person!" Tom looked around the room, catching each eye. "I mean I want you to care for me. I'm human. I like to be touched. I want a human relationship, a give-and-take. If you can tell that I care for you, don't you imagine that I can tell if you care for me?"

Tom looked at Maggie, who had a tear in her eye. "Oh, Tom."

Tom replied, "Well, we are human. We have our needs. I wonder why patients forget that." He looked over at Karen.

She was completely defused. "I hear you. I just wish I could find someone like you." She laughed, "You know, you're different."

Tom said, "Times are changing, Karen. I hope you do find a doctor who can respond to your needs."

Tom got up, signaling that he had no more to add. He patted Wendell on the shoulder. "Hold onto that friend of yours, Wendell. He sounds like a good doc to me.

Wendell shook Tom's hand. "Don't worry about that. He's one of those 9,9's, no question about it."

Tom knew that Wendell really didn't understand, but it didn't matter. In days gone by, Tom would have fulfilled Karen's expectations and ruined the evening. He knew that he had changed, and it was a good feeling.

Maggie jumped up, "Any room for dessert?"

"You bet, but only if you made it." Tom smiled as he took her hand. "Paul isn't the only one who can cook around here."

General Characteristics of the 9,9-Orientation to Medicine

This leadership style integrates high concern for medical technique with high concern for the patient, as indicated in the upper right corner of the Grid. Unlike the other medical styles, the 9,9 orientation assumes no inherent contradiction between medical technique and the human needs of patients. The 9,9-oriented physician involves all members of the medical team — including patients — in order to determine strategies of medical care based on common shared objectives. The efficiency that follows this type of teamwork has a dramatic impact on the quality of care that results.

The needs of patients are met through establishing sound, mature relationships designed to promote participation in and commitment to medical teamwork. The result is a patient who has been included from the start, has come to understand shared responsibility, has realistic expectations, and is generally satisfied, even in view of a less-than-perfect outcome.

Motivation

The motivation for 9,9 achievement is a high-spirited sense of gratification from working effectively with people and enthusiasm from making a contribution rather than fear of making a mistake. The closer one comes to reaching 9,9 medical excellence, the greater the sense of personal fulfillment. The 9,9-oriented physician embraces challenging goals, exercises diligent effort, and stimulates creative solutions to difficult medical dilemmas.

A 9,9-oriented physician's negative motivation is to avoid advancing selfish interest at the expense of patients or the medical community. To do so would invite suspicion and distrust and ultimately reduce candor in dealing with others. This physician realizes that guarded relationships impede progress and create many of the adverse conditions that are collectively called *the health care crisis.* The solution is not politics, climbing over others, contracts or formulas, withholding information, or other ways of protecting oneself at the expense of camaraderie and working together. Selfishness reduces a it self-esteem and gets in the way of true partnership, which is at the core of this medical style and what makes it the most successful of the all medical styles described in this book.

The 9,9-Oriented Physician-Patient Relationship

The 9,9-oriented physician is a solution seeker who assists patients by helping remove barriers to a successful outcome. This can only be done by placing a high value on reaching a sound medical decision that "feels right" to the patient and at the same time has the highest probability of providing the best medical outcome. This 9,9 style satisfies the patient while advancing the objective of optimal medical care.

Providing Patient Care

Participation-centered teamwork is the basis for 9,9 medical care. The patient and medical team members share responsibility with the physician for implementing truly excellent medical care. Resistance and reservations are resolved as a step towards involvement and commitment. Trust and understanding create the personal motivation for patients to work towards successful outcomes. When the entire medical team is focused on achieving medical goals that are high but realistic, and that they understand and agree with, the process becomes more meaningful and purposeful, and compliance becomes a reality. The assumption is that when individuals value the medical plan and their own real stake in carrying it out, greater reliance can be placed on self-control and self-direction. With effective leadership, patients as well as the medical team can effectively mesh their efforts.

Medical care that is 9,9 oriented rests on assumptions quite different from those previously discussed. One basic assumption is that the physician-patient relationship begins with a genuine two-sided interview. Another is that the physician becomes clear about the patient's medical problem and human needs before developing a plan for care. A third is that facts and logic are key factors in bringing about understanding of the patient's condition and a positive decision by both the physician and the patient with regard to appropriate therapy. Fourth is the view that patients are thinking people whose concerns and doubts should be dealt with fully and respectfully.

Communication. How does a physician with a 9,9 orientation go about the process of communicating that is so vital to medical excellence? The 9,9 focus is on the quality of thinking and its essential validity, regardless of whether it represents a personal view, a patient's view, or an outgrowth of their interaction. This physician may begin by reviewing the history of what is already known about the patient situation in order to clarify the patient's level of understanding. This helps to build a foundation of trust and confidence.

If, during the initial encounter, the patient seems poorly informed about the problem, the physician may begin by generally describing the benefits that reasonably can be expected from medical care. The physician defines and specifies what aspects of the patient's specific problem can be satisfied or solved with this medical plan. As the interview proceeds, the physician listens and questions to gain deeper understanding of how the care might be modified, in light of the patient's personal and emotional situation, to provide the greatest benefit.

The physician's communication style must reinforce what the physician says. The 9,9-oriented physician lets patients know they are respected as individuals and are not viewed simply as just more bodies in an assembly line of care. Other unspoken messages are that the patient's ability to think is appreciated and that the information conveyed is valued and will be used in creating a plan of care.

A prime ingredient of 9,9 communication is listening. Because this physician knows that the essence of thought and feeling is never fully captured in words, he or she is likely to repeat — not in the same words that were spoken, but according to his or her understanding of those words — the question or comment made by the patient. In this way the physician can be assured of understanding to the fullest extent possible what the patient is thinking. The 9,9-oriented physician is then in the best position to communicate with the patient in the light of real needs.

In 9,9 communication, emotions are seen as valid responses to situations being viewed objectively. A 9,9-oriented person feels antipathy toward those responsible for injustice, affection for those who are reaching out. The plight of people who are uninvolved and withdrawn is felt, and the conservative, "playing it safe" attitude of the person whose emotions are always in the middle is comprehended. Emotions provide a basis for coping self-confidently with the entire spectrum of people encountered.

This physician is able to keep personal feelings in perspective so that they do not affect the capacity to hear objectively. The aim of this physician is to help the patient to constructively find solutions to problems, at the same time realizing that a patient has unique needs, emotions, feelings, and frustrations. All these may pull conversations away from the straight path of logic. The physician sees

126

such departures not as time-consuming detours but rather as part of the art of medicine.

Establishing patient expectations. The assumption that guides the 9,9-oriented physician is that the patient can have realistic expectations about the medical care provided, even in the case of a poor outcome. For this reason, the physician works to provide an understanding of all aspects of the medical care: preevaluation testing, procedures, follow-up, and the need for compliance (cooperation). This does not mean that the physician overemphasizes medicine's limitations, but that objectivity and realism are maintained whenever limitations do exist. The following conversation exemplifies the ways in which a 9,9-oriented physician seeks to clarify expectations with a difficult patient.

Patient: It's unfortunate that you can't really guarantee your work, doctor, ha, ha! What can you promise me? I mean, it's going to be okay, isn't it?
Physician: The best answer I can give you, Jim, is that 90 percent of people with your condition recover from surgery without complications. That means one out of ten will need some additional treatment. Still, 90 percent is pretty good.
Patient: Yeah, that sounds reasonable, like everything else you say, but can you promise that something won't go wrong? History doesn't always repeat itself, you know, and I don't want to be the one with the problem because something goes wrong in the operating room.
Physician: Well, *promise* is a hard word to use. I do this procedure regularly. The hospital is a good one, and I feel sure the same equipment and conditions that have existed for the past several years will still be present next week. But, if anything does change, you have my word that I will cancel your surgery.
Patient: I expect that's about as much as I can ask. Okay. Let's get this over with. Put me on the schedule.

This patient is not yet ready to be "put on the schedule," but once the physician has gauged the patient's knowledge and dealt with this initial reservation, the interview can proceed to a more detailed discussion about the treatment and how and why it may or may not contribute to solving the patient's problems and needs. In the final analysis, it is the eye-to-eye delivery of a sense of caring for the patient that helps solidify realistic patient expectations.

Acquiring Knowledge. Heavy emphasis on fact-based solutions is one of the key features of a 9,9 medical orientation. Recognizing the persuasive power of knowledge, a 9,9-oriented physician builds self-reliance by continuous study, analysis, and inquiry regarding new medical techniques.

Studying pertinent sources in order to grasp the full complexity of the problem typifies this physician's approach. Peer review journals are examined proactively. The reader is alert and asks, "Why did the author say this? Is it a good study design?" or "That's a sweeping statement I can't let pass unchallenged." To double-check, this physician might give an article to a peer, saying, "I've reviewed this study, but I'd like to hear what you think about it."

The physician also stays well informed with regard to the patients as individuals, including their background, their experience, and the way they relate to their particular medical problem. This includes information about alternative therapies or services the patient has considered or tried, as well as the emotions of a patient. The capacity to respond to the interests, desires, and aspirations of the patient is part of acquiring knowledge.

Inquiry is comprehensive and in depth, increasing the likelihood that real problems are fully understood and that clear separation is maintained between fact and opinion. This physician has an enthusiasm for "knowing the score" that is reinforced by curiosity. Questioning becomes a two-way process, with patients and physicians equally free to ask questions of each other. Questions are basic to any inquiry, but 9,9 questions have the unique quality of being open ended. "How does this situation look to you?" "What do you know about this situation?" "When do you feel these events should take place?" "Why do you feel that way?"

Thoroughness and depth of inquiry are at the heart of 9,9 medicine. The fact that "prework is a prerequisite for participation" is another way of saying that problem solving can be no better than the thinking that leads to the conclusion, and thinking is limited by the available input of information.

Assessing the patient's needs. Although the felt needs expressed by the patient may not be the real needs, the patient's position is respected and not brushed aside. The physician's objective is to help the patient distinguish between felt and real needs if a difference exists.

The physician works to quickly establish an open, give-and-take relationship in order to facilitate exploring real needs. This is important because the subtleties of medicine always allow options, and letting the patient participate not only creates a shared involvement, but gives the physician new insight into what patients truly need.

The 9,9-oriented physician may actually come to understand the patient's problems or needs even more clearly than they are understood by the patient, who may not see them as objectively as an outside observer. The relationship that evolves is one in which two people are deliberating about how one of them can direct and the other best participate in care.

In the final analysis, the decision to accept medical care is a purchasing decision, and many times this decision is triggered by an emotional feeling of "This is what I need" based on subjective factors. The physician should acknowledge and respect this response, but realize that decisions based on logic and reason are more likely to endure than those that are solely based on impulse and emotion. This physician prefers to delay the decision until it is clear that the role of data and logic is fully acknowledged. Understanding how the decision was made reinforces the patient's emotional desires. The result is a stronger commitment to care and an increased likelihood that needs will be met.

Comparison of one's own practice with those of colleagues meets patients' needs to make a choice from a variety of options presented by several different physicians. The patient can compare and choose, making a final selection from several choices, a spectrum of costs, and differing facilities. In making this comparison, the physician demonstrates the advantages of the appropriate care without berating colleagues. This open-minded objectivity lays a foundation for building the patient's confidence in the physician and the medical plan.

The 9,9-oriented medical practice does not rest on the assumption that a set of blinders must be kept on the patient to induce acceptance of one physician's care in preference to that of another. Instead, the assumption is that when a patient can be assisted to obtain a second opinion, the physician is in a stronger position to gain confidence and respect.

If the attitude of openness and candor that typifies the 9,9-oriented physician results in a patient selecting the services of another physician, this does not mean that a 9,9 orientation is harmful to the physician's success. Indeed, if the service provided did not satisfy the particular need of the patient, this physician can then decide whether or not to take the necessary steps to improve skills in this area. Without this kind of feedback, growth is retarded and a major opportunity to continually move toward medical excellence is lost.

Decision Making. Physicians who are 9,9 oriented apply their energy to directing the appropriate medical team members toward sound decisions. This means that convictions are developed and expressed, and reservations are discussed in a direct, logical, and convincing manner. This approach is balanced with human understanding and, as a result, the 9,9-oriented physician earns wide respect for his or her convictions, opinions, and values. This readiness to advocate positions may result in this physician being seen as self-assured and strong-willed, but openness to alternative points of view negates any feeling of rigidity.

Decisions are reached after thorough inquiry and advocacy. As a result, decisions become a natural outgrowth of a process rather than the physician's unilateral conclusion issued as an ultimatum.

When a decision involves several people, 9,9 decision making seeks understanding and agreement among all participants, whether they include the patient, family, or medical team members. The coupling of the words *understanding* and *agreement* is important, because action without understanding can be little more than obedience and may therefore constitute a barrier to cooperation.

Within the medical team, 9,9 cooperation can follow several patterns in that it would be unrealistic to expect everyone to be involved in making decisions all of the time. As an example, patients may have nothing to contribute to the solution of a technical problem and may not be specifically involved in implementing it. For them to take part is a misuse of their role. Although 9,9 decision making in no way reduces the hierarchical authority and responsibility of the physician to achieve results, all decisions can be thought of in terms of team dynamics. Let's review who actually participates in medical problem solving during a variety of typical encounters.

One-alone. In the interest of productive use of human resources, the one-alone (1/0) pattern of decision making is used when one member has the responsibility, the capacity, and the information to solve the problem. That person solves the problem alone and then lets others know how the solution affects their own responsibilities. Individual effectiveness contributes to teamwork by moving the team toward its goal and avoiding duplication of effort.

One-to-one. Problems that involve the physician and any one of the other team members working together can be grouped as one-to-one (1/1) team actions. Occasionally a pair works out the solution and takes actions that move the team toward its goals. A common example is the one-to-one decisions made between the physician and the consultant. When these 1/1 actions occur between a physician and another member of the team, they are traditionally thought of as a process of delegation.

This orientation to decision making has important implications for training as well as practice. The physician aids those consulted to gain experiences that increase their autonomy and sense of achievement. This type of delegation frees the physician for other activities, but it also creates a new level of understanding.

One 9,9-oriented physician described her approach to 1/1 decision making this way:

"With nurses or residents who have less experience, I identify the problem and discuss it with them. I ask them to develop an approach to doing the task, much as I would with any consultant. Then I review their thinking to see if I can contribute to unsolved problems before encouraging the next step.

"After experience has been developed, I ask those who have questions to review plans and solutions with their colleagues and to come to me only when a solution cannot be found or when a shift in direction is called for. Getting help and critique from colleagues is critical to successful delegation and development. I remain responsible and available when problems cannot be resolved by the team."

Through this process, the physician-to-team-member activities that are 1/1 in character are reviewed by all members of the team for their additional contributions as well as for cross-learning through critique. The key is that 1/1 situations can involve any team member interacting with any other member according to each it specific area of responsibility and need for input.

One-to-one-to-one. This pattern is also critical to medical decision making. A member takes a certain action that makes it possible for another member to take a subsequent action and so on until all necessary steps are taken to achieve the end result. Each team member's contribution is indispensable to a successful sequence. For example, when a physician writes an order, a complex sequence of interdependent operations begins. Smooth coordination is needed between the physician and those who receive the order, those who carry it out, the patient who must cooperate, and the family who must support the patient. Done well, this coordinated effort satisfies the patient and builds trust and the best possible medical outcomes. Though few face-to-face meetings may take place, each team member's contribution links them together in the effort.

One-to-some. Here medical care involves more than two people but not the total team. The pattern falls between 1/1 and 1/all, and what differs is the number of members involved rather than whether actions are simultaneous or sequential. Therefore, the pattern is not considered separately here. It is characterized only as a reminder that one-to-some interactions are utilized when needed.

One-to-all. Some decisions can only be made by all members of the team working together. Such one-to-all (1/all) problems bring together everyone involved in achieving a common purpose or in dealing with a given problem that touches on everyone.

Decision making that is 1/all occurs when 1) no team member has enough knowledge, information, or expertise to formulate the total answer, but everyone working together can be expected to reach it; 2) coordination of each member's participation is significant to a successful outcome; and 3) all must understand the overall effort so that each takes responsibility for his or her contribution to the final outcome. This type of decision making is becoming more common due to the addition of allied health care providers and graduate level nurses to what were already complex clinical teams.

Level of responsibility. Because 9,9 decision making rests on stimulating the involvement of patients, a final decision about medical care is recommended only when the patient takes an active role in the process. Understanding and agreement between physician and patient are reinforced by mutual feelings that the decision is the right one. The physician acts as the leader in establishing a climate of give-and-take. This is done by exploring the patient's actual needs and how these can best be satisfied within the limits acknowledged by both parties.

Limits include the imperfections of medicine and budgetary restraints set by the patient. Within these boundaries, a sound medical plan can usually be developed that is satisfactory from the point of view of each party. The level of responsibility is ideal when the patient is involved in arriving at a decision to participate in a plan that truly satisfies realistic needs.

Initiative. Initiative that is 9,9 oriented is exercised in a strong manner. The physician is likely to be eager, vigorous, and able to sustain a significant capacity for work.

The 9,9-oriented physician sets priorities and then follows through, retesting along the way to ensure soundness. Two problems may be equally important but not equally urgent. If two problems have the same significance and the same urgency, the one with the higher likelihood of good results takes priority. If two equally good results are expected, the one that can be completed with less time and expense gets priority.

Also, initiative that is 9,9 oriented is exercised as a part of medical team membership. Widespread and spontaneous initiative-taking ensures that no one will say, "That's not my problem; I'm not the physician." This physician initiates actions through other people so that patients and medical team members accept responsibility in carrying out the medical plan.

Conflict Resolution. An error that many physicians make is assuming that conflict occurs only at the point of anger, total misunderstanding, or absolute refusal to work together. In reality, conflicts are those differences of opinion that constitute a part of everyday communication. Because conflicts are linked to the subjective element of people's behavior, physicians often neglect conflicts as they try to understand medical dilemmas. Physicians who are 9,9 oriented see conflict as a warning signal that some concern of the patient or medical team member has not been adequately resolved.

The following skills allow 9,9-oriented physicians to have disagreements that can be resolved without creating animosity.

Getting early involvement. Involving others early in problems that affect them provides the opportunity for gathering additional information and also allows alternatives to be identified. Faulty logic and distorted perspectives can be recognized and dealt with, and, most importantly, incorrect information can be eliminated. Each of these steps decreases the likelihood of mistakes and misunderstanding.

Full self-disclosure within the framework of medical care. Self-disclosure is complete when everything that bears directly on the medical situation, including data, logic, attitudes, feelings, hunches, and even intuition, has been discussed at length.

Developing criteria. Getting agreement on the elements of a sound solution before searching for an actual solution is an excellent way of avoiding conflict and of getting better results. When two people use shared criteria to evaluate the soundness of a solution, disagreement is unlikely to shift into armed conflict.

Handling Conflict When It Appears

Confrontation. Many physicians dread confrontation, but it can be used to an advantage in attaining medical excellence. The word *confrontation* has two distinct meanings, and because there is no good substitute for this term, it is important to distinguish between them.

One meaning of confrontation rests upon the concept of bringing opposing points of view into sharp focus as a means of testing one's strength against another's. The underlying assumption is that one it view will prevail over the other. This is confrontation as combat, and it is the 9,1 approach to ending differences.

Confrontation as comparison and contrast has quite a different meaning. It rests on solving conflict by focusing on differences. When conflict is brought out into the open and differences are discussed, those who are a party to them can resolve them directly. Emotions that usually accompany conflict — anger, hostility, fear, anxiety, doubt, and disappointment — can also be dealt with.

Viewed by an observer, confrontation as combat and confrontation as comparison and contrast might appear similar. However, an important underlying difference is easily recognized by those individuals engaged in the confrontation. In the case of confrontation as combat, there is a contest of wills. The holder of one view feels threatened by the holder of the other. To yield in this kind of confrontation means being forced by one's own weakness to accept the other position. Karen's goal in her battle with Dr. Jones at the dinner party was to win.

The meaning of confrontation as comparison and contrast implies mutual trust and a desire for understanding among those who are trying to resolve the difference. Trust implies goodwill, good intentions, and respect for others — whether they agree or disagree. For either viewpoint to prevail over the other is unimportant. Out of comparison and contrast, a position may emerge that incorporates something of both viewpoints but also adds elements of uniqueness, inclusiveness, and so forth, that make it superior to either. Another possibility is that an entirely different solution will be found. Finding a sound solution is the key concept that leads to medical excellence, yet the process by which this can be accomplished has been one of the most difficult for physicians to adopt.

Being open minded, considering alternatives, testing consequences, and being forthright are all critical in seeking sound solutions. Under these conditions, one it yielding to the position of another is not capitulation. It entails no loss of face; it is no measure of weakness. Rather, it is a demonstration of commitment to a best solution achieved through logic and reason and the removal of reservations and doubts.

The two meanings of confrontation can be distinguished simply and clearly: The first meaning is based on answering the question, "Who is right?" The second is, "What is right?" The answer to that question provides growth and a type of feedback that is essential to developing relationships that lead to sound medical plans.

Dealing with patient objections. Almost invariably patients raise doubts and reservations when hearing a medical plan for the first time. Recognizing this fact, the 9,9-oriented physician creates opportunities for the patient to express and discuss misgivings throughout the interview. The physician knows that if these are not brought out, they are likely to persist and to influence the patient's thinking and feelings adversely. When these doubts are expressed openly, the physician can respond to them and remove them as barriers to high-quality care.

There are several kinds of reservations. Some result from a lack of information. In these cases, the physician seeks to understand the patient's views by asking supplementary questions to clarify what information is needed. Only then is the physician in a position to dissolve initial objections and to gain support for the ongoing relationship.

Other objections may be based on misinformation about the limitations of a procedure or its statistical success rate. The physician then invites the patient to participate in examining these issues, thus creating an opportunity to find out what the misunderstandings actually are. Misinformation can then be replaced by valid information that eliminates the objection.

Sometimes unstated objections are founded upon reservations and doubts rooted solely in the patient's feelings. The patient is often quite unaware that emotions are affecting personal objectivity. By encouraging the patient to express feelings about the medical plan and listening attentively to what is said, the physician may come to understand what is bothering the patient. If the physician is genuinely trying to bring out the patient's reservations and objections for discussion, rather than looking for ammunition to win arguments, the patient will usually recognize the honest motivation and respect the physician for it.

The following dialogue, begun by the physician, illustrates a 9,9 approach to dealing with reservations and objections:

Physician: What other questions do you have?
Patient: Well, there is one. Isn't this treatment likely to be out of date within a year or so? Innovations are coming along so fast that a better treatment is likely to appear just about the same time I am recovering from the side effects of this one, don't you think?

Physician: The rate of medical advancement seems to accelerate each year, but I am not expecting any major advances in treating your disease.

Patient: But it could happen, so maybe I should postpone making a decision. This is my life we are talking about.

Physician: I know you need this treatment, and I'd like to see you have it, but I certainly respect your feelings. What if the situation is the same next year?

Patient: Well, I don't know.

Physician: What do you mean?

Patient: (silence)

Physician: The fact is that this disease progresses gradually; you know it keeps getting worse. The approach to treatment will undergo minor changes, but several years usually pass between major innovations. This particular treatment is based on the latest technology, so significant improvements will probably not appear for a good number of years. Minor modifications will be made, but until years of data have been collected, it's always hard to say if they are better or worse than what is currently in use. So why don't you weigh the risks and the benefits of starting therapy now? The medical plan that we've developed has a lot of thought behind it. My feeling is that it is very likely to be what you need.

Patient: Yeah, it all makes sense. I just hate having this problem; it's not fair. But I'll think about what you've said.

Physician: At least there are steps you and I can take together to put up a good fight.

When a patient's objection is based on valid reasoning, the 9,9 approach is to acknowledge the objection and then to openly explore realistic possibilities for dealing conclusively with it. This may involve probing in order to get to the root of the patient's thinking. More often than not, when an objection or disagreement is discussed candidly, one of two things occurs. Either it turns out to be less important than it first appeared, or creative ways can be found for modifying the plan to more fully address the patient's needs and still ensure top medical-technical care.

The 9,9 orientation is based on the assumption that valid ends have a greater likelihood of being reached when valid means to those ends are employed. Thus, integrity is basic to the 9,9 orientation. Truth is sought through an openness and candor that acknowledge existing limitations. If attempts have already been made to clarify any incorrect information through a process of sharing perspectives, if full disclosure within the framework of the medical care has been achieved, if the communication has been clear, and if effort was applied to developing criteria for resolving the conflict, and the conflict still persists, then additional steps will need to be taken.

Ventilation is a technique that can be used by either the physician or the patient to discuss frustrations and discouraging issues with a third party. Sometimes this technique reduces tension sufficiently for increased efforts at problem solving to take place.

Review and feedback from an uninvolved third party may also be of benefit. Disagreeing parties may be so enmeshed in the problem that they have lost objectivity and need a new perspective. The "neutral" individual may be another physician, a nurse, or a consultant — anyone who has no vested interest in the outcome.

When all else fails and the conflict persists, but high-quality medical care is critical to the patient's well-being, the 9,9-oriented physician is faced with a difficult decision. Moving to medical care when objections are unresolved carries medical-legal risks, but the alternative is resignation and that is seldom an acceptable course to this physician. Suggesting that the patient seek a second opinion or offering to refer the patient to another competent physician may be preferable solutions.

Critique and Feedback. Hoping to learn from experience and to ensure the highest quality medical care, this physician reviews each failure as well as each success, critiquing why the effort went well or why it did not. Lack of success with one patient may provide insight into how to achieve better results with the next. This is one source of the resilience that characterizes the 9,9-oriented physician.

This physician has an open mind and is continually searching for ways to enhance strategies that work well and, by trying to comprehend the inexplicable in each medical situation, to discover new ones. This physician realizes that analyzing a success frequently contributes more useful knowledge toward achieving medical excellence than taking the traditional approach of analyzing problems. Continuous examination ensures that all steps in the process are as effective as possible.

No one is likely to be in the unique position of making the sole contribution to critique and feedback by virtue of rank or even experience. The 9,9-oriented physician is self-critical and receptive to feedback from others. When critique is effective, the potential for strengthened decisions is great. The double-loop approach to feedback permits growth to occur.

The effectiveness of critique is characterized by properties such as the following:

- Openness and candor prevail because all members of the medical team recognize that these foster the "best decisions."
- Critique occurs throughout medical care, not just at special points along the way or as a postmortem that reconstructs the history of the case.
- One aspect of critique describes what has happened and the consequences that resulted, and therefore is undertaken as soon as possible after the case occurs so that the cause-and-effect relationship is clear.
- While critique analyzes the consequences of actions, it tacitly avoids

valuative judgments of good or bad, right or wrong.

- Critique considers connections between personal behavior and consequences. However, social topics and personal observations are only pertinent insofar as they relate to delivering care. Outside matters such as politics, religion, social engagements, and friendships have no real pertinence and are out of bounds.

Barriers to effectiveness arise from many sources, and no one of them is more or less important than any other, because all can impede sound decision making. The most common of these barriers are faulty logic, vested interest, hidden agendas, jealousies, favoritism, blindness to options, fear-provoking remarks, poor timing, unwitting acceptance of low-caliber goals, and overlooked contributions. If these barriers are not overcome, they will always limit the quality of care that is achieved.

Informed consent. The 9,9 approach to informed consent is often a foregone conclusion to the physician-patient interview, because reservations and doubts have been identified, discussed, and resolved along the way. An essential feature of informed consent is summing up, which is a part of critique and feedback. This is not the loaded machine-gun summary of benefits that many physicians employ, nor is it a bold statement of pros and cons that leaves patients feeling uncertain about the plan for care. The 9,9 orientation to informed consent aids the patient in crystallizing his or her thinking and in weighing the decision in the light of all the points previously developed.

The fact that both the patient and physician are working toward a mutual goal permits the patient to pose any additional inquiries. Although further reservations and doubts are not encouraged, the patient is provided the opportunity to identify ones that may not yet have been expressed.

Research and experience support the conclusion that physician-patient interviews conducted in a 9,9 orientation are most likely to pass through the various steps in the sequence and to reach true informed consent. When easy rapport has been established, a friendly give-and-take quickly leads to an effective analysis of the patient's needs. The needs analysis penetrates the expressed needs and identifies the real needs that underlie the patient's motivation for coming to see the physician in the first place. The interview is functional in the sense that it balances medical limitations with real patient needs and discovers the optimum fit.

Nothing beyond simple mechanics remains to be completed at the point of true informed consent, and these matters are carried to conclusion in a supportive atmosphere of shared responsibility. The physician is pleased to have brought the patient into a collaborative relationship and to have facilitated a sound decision. The patient is satisfied because personal convictions expressed in making the decision are self-reinforcing.

New and Established Patients

In order to accomplish the high level of informed consent and to secure shared responsibility, this physician is dedicated to establishing a physician-patient relationship based on trust and mutual respect. This is a time-consuming objective, and interviews are likely to be lengthy, particularly for new patients and for established patients who develop serious conditions. Patients need to sense that they have the physician's undivided attention and that their concerns are valid. A basis for communication can then be established.

Challenging situations exist when the patient is faced with a life-threatening problem or appears indifferent during the initial explanation of a treatment plan that is critical to care. In these cases the 9,9-oriented physician seeks to understand and break down the barrier — whether it is fear or resignation — to establishing an open partnership. What the physician has to say is both purposeful and authentic, setting the keynote of frankness for a productive discussion.

The physician is alert to the individual needs of new patients. From the beginning the physician is self-assured but not arrogant, reassuring the patient by his or her attitude and expertise. The physician begins to develop an information bank through a sincere interest in the patient's needs and objectives, which encourages the patient's active involvement and participation. The 9,9-oriented physician establishes a pace that takes into consideration the patient's readiness to focus attention on the real problem to be solved. Whether a physician is acting in the patient's best interest or whether the real aim is to keep the patients moving through the office becomes readily apparent to the patient.

When the interview has been brought to a successful end, an excellent foundation has been laid for encouraging the patient's ongoing involvement in health care. This physician impacts the patient in a way that makes him or her responsive to future medical care. The patient is likely to consult the physician when confronted with any medical problem in the belief that the physician is a trustworthy resource. This type of relationship leads not only to a successful practice, but also to a patient who takes responsibility for his or her own health.

Coping with the Busy Practice

The 9,9-oriented physician will be in demand and will be faced with the challenge of a busy practice. This offers increasing monetary reward, but the problems in a very busy practice are twofold: Competitors who are able to satisfy the patient's need in a more timely manner may usurp this doctor's business, and while it may be possible to squeeze people in as a means of avoiding delays, this solution is incompatible with this physician's practice style.

Because this physician stays with problems until each patient is satisfied and the highest quality care has been achieved, or until the possibility of serving the patient has become unrealistic, alternative solutions to patient volume may need to be considered. Paramedical personnel may be hired to lighten the load, often resulting in no personal profit to the physician. A simpler solution may be to see fewer patients, the physician's personal satisfaction from achieving excellence outweighing the decrease in income.

The following quotes may be helpful in seeing how the 9,9-oriented physician copes with his or her practice:

Scheduling and Time Management. "I put effort into scheduling my activities to meet my practice objectives. In this way I can fulfill all of my responsibilities and respond to emergencies as they arise. When I formulate a sound plan, I follow it from start to completion unless a sounder plan emerges. Because I gather the reactions of patients and the medical team on an ongoing basis, the goals that I establish reflect the concerns of my team."

The Hospital. "Work requirements are matched with personal capabilities or needs within the medical team. Together, we determine individual responsibilities, procedures, and ground rules. In addition to ongoing critiques designed to keep care running smoothly, we conduct reviews of care. Evaluating how things went permits us to see what we have learned and how we can apply it to future situations. I give recognition to the medical team, and the team recognizes outstanding individual contributions."

Expenses. "The expenses under my control are essential for conducting my business, and my integrity and prudence provide guidance as I incur them. Full value in terms of patient satisfaction is realized from the money I spend. The amount of money I require as profit is in balance with obtaining security and enjoying a pleasant and rewarding life style."

Continuing Education. "By analyzing reasons for failures as well as successes, I improve my skills and increase my professional contribution. I seek to understand how and why patients respond in the ways that they do to the stress that illness puts upon them. I review medical techniques and update my fund of knowledge to a point where I am comfortable with the medical advice that I give. I also study human resources, teamwork, and communication techniques so that I am effective and seldom misunderstood."

Self-Evaluation. "My criteria for evaluating my own performance are worked out at the beginning of a medical care plan, and the concrete indicators of success are specified in advance. The patient and medical team members provide another perspective by offering and receiving feedback and critique. Once past performance has been appraised, new objectives for the next situation are established with concrete indicators of progress. I am ready to proceed with care, once again applying this framework for assessing the patient involvement and my own role in reaching the best possible outcome."

Recognizing 9,9 Behavior

Before considering the physician-patient relationship, it may be helpful to review simple words and phrases that describe 9,9 behavior:

Candid and forthright
Clear about priorities
Confident
Decisive
Determined
Enjoys working
Fact finder
Focuses on real issues
Follows through
Gets issues into the open
Has a "can do" spirit
Has high standards
Identifies underlying causes
Innovative
Open minded
Positive
Reflective
Sets challenging goals
Spontaneous
Stands ground
Stimulates participation
Straight shooter
Unselfish

Patient Reactions Based On Grid Styles

A 9,9 orientation has a greater likelihood of achieving high-quality results with difficult patients than any other Grid style. This is because 9,9-oriented assumptions provide a valid basis for accommodating the physician's recommendation to the patient's real needs. The goal here is to achieve 9,9-oriented reactions from every patient, regardless of the patient's natural Grid style.

9,1

The 9,9-oriented physician's high concern for the patient's problem is compatible with the 9,1-oriented patient's objective of getting good care, although this physician cannot be pressured into unjustifiable concessions. Being open and aboveboard prevents suspicion and tends to reduce unwarranted fears of being "taken advantage of." The physician is simultaneously responsive to the 9,1-oriented patient's objective of "getting the most the system will allow" and to the defensive posture toward making a decision of "show me" or "prove it to me." The physician anticipates that this patient will act in a provocative manner and will have negative, skeptical attitudes.

The 9,9 response to the 9,1-oriented patient is patience, realizing the first point of entry is to develop trust by providing general background knowledge. Then some easy questions are introduced in such a way that they do not place pressure on the patient to admit ignorance but capture interest by stimulating the patient to think constructively. Queries and negative reactions provide the physician with various clues as to what additional information is required. Next, the physician elicits descriptions of what the patient hopes to accomplish.

By getting the patient to consider knowledge and desires simultaneously, the physician develops a basis for making sure that the patient's expectations are in concert with realistic possibilities. 9,9-oriented physicians rarely allow even this patient to place them in the position of fighting back in a win-lose battle. However, if this occurs, the 9,9-oriented approach is to find out the real reason for the resentment and to work for a solution that prevents it from becoming a problem again.

These difficult patients are eager to learn but often have had a bad experience somewhere along the road to medical care. When trust is reestablished, they can become patients who are dedicated and are relieved to have found a physician they did not think existed.

1,9

A 9,9-oriented physician's approach meets the 1,9-oriented patient's desire to be liked, but the physician quickly senses the risks inherent in a swift and easy physician-patient encounter. As the result of involving the patient in reaching a sound decision, a new level of trust and respect for this physician can be established. If that cannot be accomplished, the patient will remain difficult, because he or she wants the physician to take full responsibility for the medical outcome.

Rather than starting with a knowledge-based presentation, the physician begins by probing the 1,9-oriented patient's feelings as a means of gaining a deeper understanding of the patient's needs. The physician often finds that the patient's desires are based more on emotions than on realistic assessments. The tasks then are to supplement the patient's knowledge and to identify and counter any unrealistic expectations. These patients are difficult until they acquire the necessary knowledge to participate in the decision-making process. So the physician provides facts and data, but the language is tailored to the patient's level of sophistication and listening skills are high to ensure that the patient understands.

Because a 1,9-oriented patient is prepared to accept whatever information is provided, the physician tests continuously to make sure that the patient has not passed the point of saturation, that true comprehension exists, and that each additional point is being related to what has been explained previously.

When 1,9-oriented patients are faced with a decision, personal involvement and participation by supportive family members, rather than logic, are used to arouse their interest and to develop genuine convictions. In this way the 9,9-oriented physician can bring even 1,9-oriented patients to a decision based on genuine understanding of evidence. These patients will be uncomfortable with the challenge of learning so much new information but, looking back, they will take pride in the shared accomplishments.

1,1

The 9,9-oriented physician approach focuses on activating a back-up style in the dominantly 1,1-oriented patient and on stimulating an otherwise dormant interest in care. Efforts to overcome 1,1 apathy are manifest in the way the physician works to discover anything that sparks interest in the patient. Initial inquiries are limited in scope and aimed at eliciting simple answers. The objective is to evoke a response or to locate a foundation of understanding to build on in order to successfully provide medical care. When faced with silence, physical contact may be used to build a link to this patient. Because 1,1 is not a natural style, the physician attempts to discover where these patients have come from and why they are now acting 1,1. Once that is clear, a new approach can be used that may work with that style.

These patients tend to miss the real opportunity modern medicine offers, but this physician stands the best chance of getting them back into the system.

5,5

The 5,5-oriented patient is responsive to this physician because the patient is treated as a person worthy of respect. The physician is not overly solicitous, but the patient is inspired to be involved. Being knowledgeable about alternatives available in the community, the physician steers the patient's thinking along problem-solving channels, ferreting out real needs from the need to do what is "in" at that particular moment. The 9,9 approach is to convert the patient's customary reliance on reputation and prestige into a greater readiness to consider innovative and creative solutions. When these patients can see how a proposed plan fits their actual needs, tentativeness changes to a sound basis for action. The physician bolsters confidence by helping the patient gain insight into how the medical plan will take shape and how the treatment will meet personal desires and ensure the highest quality outcome possible.

9,9

The greatest personal reward for the 9,9-oriented physician is delivering care to a 9,9-oriented patient. The approach clicks immediately with such a patient. Not only is the interview geared to responding to the patient's real needs, but it clearly depends on fact-based logical reasoning. Efforts are made to ensure that the patient's expectations about the medical plan are realistic and valid. From then on, patient and physician become consultants to one another as to the soundest actions to take. The physician follows valid principles for creating conditions for the patient's participation in problem solving, and a shared and successful outcome is the most likely result. The physician possesses great strength based on an in-depth knowledge of medical techniques; the result is solutions that fit the patient's human needs to participate in his or her own life.

The importance of realistic expectations regarding what the medical plan will or will not accomplish is equally clear to both the physician and the patient. Through a natural process of give-and-take, both search to define realistic and valid expectations, knowing that these are the foundation for making sound decisions. Limitations can be discussed openly, without fear that this discussion might itself be a reason for litigation if a poor outcome results.

This combination is estimated to make up less than 5% of medical relationships, yet it is the most rewarding and safest place to practice medicine today. Another way to state this is that 95% of the time care is being provided to difficult patients or the physician is using one of the other grid styles. The goal then is to move patients toward the 9,9 style, and the 9,9 approach has the greatest potential to meet this challenge.

Summary

The 9,9-oriented physician understands the complex and subtle factors that enter into ensuring medical excellence. This physician does not automatically assume that nothing should be allowed to stand in the way of medical care, as is likely to be true for a 9,1 orientation, or that no patient request is unreasonable, as a 1,9 orientation might suggest. Rather, the attitude is, "My goal is satisfying patients' needs while adhering to the highest medical standard. I do this by providing good medical care with full patient understanding. This approach is in the best long-term interest of my profession, my patient, and myself."

All things considered, a 9,9 orientation runs the fewest risks of poor-quality medical outcome, particularly when viewed in a long-term perspective. It brings the greatest possible benefits to the patient, as well as ensuring patient satisfaction. This approach, which encompasses not only medical-technical excellence but meeting human needs in a time of life crisis, takes physicians into a new era in which the healing hand, which was once the only tool for physicians, is integrated with tremendous technology, which is literally capable of producing medical miracles. In this sense, the potential rewards for practicing medicine have never been greater, yet a 9,9 orientation to the rapid and radical changes that face medical practice is the only strategy that stands to give physicians the heightened sense of fulfillment they deserve.

Chapter Ten

INTEGRATING CLINICAL PRACTICE IMPROVEMENT AND RISK MANAGEMENT: MEETING THE NEEDS OF THE DIFFICULT PATIENT

Understanding the various Grid styles and what your most dominant style is are the first steps needed to build a strategy that will ensure the highest quality care by meeting all of your patients' needs. Focusing on litigation as a barometer of patient satisfaction may have limitations, but the realities of medical practice today require that it be done, in addition to evaluating quality.

Systems of care are emerging under the financial influence of increased competition and provider at risk reimbursement. The systems that will help you meet even the difficult patient's needs cannot be based on compromise and cookbook medicine, because the distance to fall from this "safe" practice to medical misadventure is so short. The new systems we are joining in record numbers must alleviate the frustrations of care providers in order to avert the ever higher tendency toward resignation and, for some, even leaving the field of medicine. To say that the best systems will rest on the creation of 9,9-oriented physicians and 9,9-oriented patients may sound like an unattainable ideal, and to assume that this goal is feasible with all patients and all physicians is unrealistic. Yet this level of aspiration leaves room for fluctuations to occur in response to the various stresses of life, and, at the very least, 5,5 care can be provided as a fall-back position. For the sake of our profession, it is time for physicians to take the lead and insist on these basic principles as components of our model of medical care.

At 39,000 Feet

The belief that this approach to improve performance can be successfully implemented in medicine was based on the precedent of another group of highly respected, highly trained professionals who had come under fire, despite the fact that they have been demanding excellence of themselves through a period of highly technological change. Technological advances in the aviation industry have revolutionized the thinking process of the world. The professional at the helm, the captain, the pilot, has moved beyond the days of experimental aircraft to a position of prominence in a highly mobile, global society. The number of technical errors compared to air time has steadily decreased through the use of highly sophisticated equipment and rigorous training programs, yet public dissatisfaction with the air industry, similar to the disenchantment with medicine, has never been higher.

In 1979, the National Aeronautics and Space Administration published a study that revealed the causes of airline industry accidents and near accidents. The gist of their conclusions is paraphrased in the following statement:

> Too many crashes and near misses occur in circumstances where the "ultimate cause" cannot be traced to air-to-ground communications, equipment failure, lack of technical competence, or a time factor. In too many cases, it has been demonstrated that adequate technical resources for solving the problem *were available* in the cockpit, but were not mobilized effectively.(1)

What was needed was enhanced communication and teamwork, and the analogies between the approach United Airlines took toward the development of their highly effective Cockpit Resource Management program and the medical resource management approach that is now being implemented in health care delivery systems are fascinating. Rather than reviewing the intricacies of this development process, we will highlight the major issues and allow you to draw your own conclusions as to their applicability to your role as a physician.

At the beginning of program development, the cockpit crew made a major point with regard to the exercise of captain authority. They emphasized decisiveness as an indispensable component of leadership. Without decisiveness, uncertainty might be communicated, allowing for divergent, uncoordinated, individually centered actions. At the extreme, a condition for insubordination might even be created. Their concerns mirror those of a physician feeling the need to ensure a rigid process for carrying out orders that have been written in the hospital chart. A primary goal, therefore, was that captain authority be maintained so that conditions favorable to insubordination were not created. In any high-stress, hazardous setting, whether the leader is commanding a highly sophisticated jet aircraft or performing the most technically advanced medical procedure, crises can and all too frequently do occur. When an emergency situation develops, the leader's response is a critical factor in determining the likelihood of a desirable and safe outcome. The typical airline captain's response to a crisis is 9,1; dominating, mastering, and controlling the situation by quickly announcing the course of action to be implemented. When the crisis has been averted, 9+9 appreciation for dutiful compliance is often extended. While this response is certainly decisive, and an approach that has been traditionally accepted and taught, research indicates that it is not always the best response. In some instances, immediate unilateral action taken by the captain without the opportunity for other crew members to add information or to suggest alternatives has proven not only ineffective but deadly.

In contrast to this response, the 9,9 orientation to leadership in the same hazardous situations remains consistent with the principles of openness, participation, and contribution. After soliciting others' ideas, recommendations, and reservations, the leader develops the soundest possible definition of the problem and proceeds quickly to a solution. The key is mobilizing all available resources to address the problem at hand and then applying the same skills of decisiveness that at one point were wasted on authoritarian rule. The results speak for themselves.

To this point, over 7,000 airline industry captains, first officers, and flight engineers have learned this 9,9-oriented approach to crew leadership and teamwork. Simulator studies reveal that such learning enhances the quality of solutions to programmed crises that are unexpected by the crew, thereby increasing the likelihood that in-flight emergencies will also be resolved safely. Additionally, "United crew members have had a 50 percent lower mistake rate on FAA proficiency checks than they did before the program was started."[2] On the basis of these results, United Airlines is the first airline company to have obtained an exemption from the Federal Aviation Administration that reduces the requirement for recurrent training by one day per pilot per year. Not only has the program proved effective, it has also resulted in significant savings in the costs associated with pilot training.

Several major airlines have established programs similar to this one as part of their training requirements, and some have already benefitted financially. In its role as liability insurance carrier for an Asian airline, Lloyds of London has provided reductions in insurance rates because the cockpit crews have completed this program. Ongoing reports detailing the experiences of other airlines continue to verify that human error and inability to effectively mobilize available technology are significant factors in airline crashes.

Another benefit of this program is the personal issue that pilots themselves take less of a risk every time they fly. This point is particularly important, as it provides hope for physicians involved in the new practice of medicine. Professional survival in an era of medical-legal crisis and utilization profiles requires insurability. The result of a poor litigation record is that liability insurance is in jeopardy. With inadequate insurance, physicians risk entire financial estates, potentially the reward for a lifetime of work. The impact of quality assurance data comparisons may also be an issue if those physicians in the bottom half of all physicians practicing are seen as a liability to the hospital or group practice collecting the data.

The incentive for pilots to take this educational program is to exceed their already high standards, and the crisis that now exists in medicine has provided the same stimulus for physicians. The sound steps that will create the kind of teamwork necessary to reach and implement a 9,9 solution are possible because the team uses a common nonthreatening language based on a theory that is accepted by all team members.

Even though the suggestions that follow continue to focus on the physician as the key figure of responsibility, 9,9 teamwork will require that entire integrated delivery systems start working together under dynamically improving models of health care delivery. The processes of care will be measured as well as outcomes. Where this model has been put in place, outcome improvements as well as liability risks have been impressive.

The Practical Steps to Integrating Clinical Practice Improvement and Risk Management

A good title for your effort is simply clinical practice improvement (CPI), but a logical approach is to structure it around the six elements of leadership: communication, acquiring knowledge, decision making, initiating an action, resolving conflict, and utilizing critique and feedback in a positive and constructive manner. The easiest way to think of this program is in terms of your "new" career of medicine, a career that you are in charge of creating.

The problem with careers, in general, is that sometimes they get out of hand. At times we all feel like victims of whatever job situation we find ourselves in. Certainly physicians are no exception. You did not predict the medical malpractice crisis or the emergence of managed care, both of which make profitability more challenging. Perhaps you are in a large practice under strict contracts and, because of that, feel the same pressures as any highly skilled "employee." Whether you are self-employed, a partner in a group practice, or an employee of a large corporation, your career is still your decision, and the controls you have over it may surprise you.

Luckily, there are experts in the world who have dedicated their lives to helping you not only understand your career, but ensure that it is as enjoyable and rewarding as possible. Richard N. Bolles may head the list in making what individuals "do for a living" practical and, most important, enjoyable. Many of the ideas briefly outlined in this chapter are patterned after work that he has spent a fair portion of his life refining. His books, *What Color Is Your Parachute?*(3) and *The Three Boxes of Life*(4), are the best practical texts we know for the true career changer. We are not suggesting you get out of medicine, but the field of medicine has changed around you. You will now have to change many aspects of your career, or someone will change your career for you.

The Issues

Successes will come to those who can organize professional principles into a competitive infrastructure where physicians can access the information they need to improve medical care. Basic issues to ensuring high-quality care in even the most difficult situations are that of shared responsibility and being able to meet the human needs of both patients and other professionals. An underlying question to direct your efforts is, "What are the medical issues that my particular practice deals with?" Rather than trying to outline them all, focus on those that are hard for patients to understand or are repeatedly involved in lawsuits. In general, life-threatening diagnoses, emergencies, surgical procedures, and any situation resulting in long-term disability are good places to start. You can actually list the major medical issues around which you and your colleagues will build your 9,9 medical philosophy and the new system of care we have been discussing. Once you have defined the medical issues, six areas of concern will carry equal value as you move to a new way to practice. These six areas are reviewed in the next section of this chapter. They are special knowledge, people, location, working conditions, level of responsibility/budget, and objectives-goals-values.

Special Knowledge

Medical Technology

The medical-technical expertise that will always be the base on which to build your system of care program arises from your training in the field of medicine and a new understanding of statistical analysis and community-based clinical trials. Your specialty board's standards will increasingly be the rule by which you are measured in a court of law. The standards were originally used as encouragement to physicians to expand their horizons or move into new areas. Unfortunately, they have now been targeted as "the minimum standard" required of physicians to avoid accusations of malpractice.

The next wave of excellent care will build new "community standards for medical-technical expertise." These standards lie within your specific hospital or medical group. The new system of care will use proven clinical practice improvement methods to document best care at the lowest necessary cost. When circumstances don't allow for improvement, a standard approach matched to the working diagnosis remains the logical fall-back position.

The Elements of Leadership

The six elements of clinical leadership described in this text are essential if we are to successfully create a new system of care. As far as communication, the team is obligated to hear what the patient says and to help the patient understand the complex clinical information through the use of a simple language. In the area of acquiring knowledge, the lost opportunity that can result when the alternative diagnoses and therapies are not addressed needs to be avoided. Thorough attention to all available data, including process data, has become a requirement to achieve new levels of excellence. Once a point of decision making has been reached, logical, scientific reasoning is the hallmark of sound medical judgment. A decision that reflects the data can change majority opinion and is generally wiser than hanging onto past practices. Initiation, too, is patterned on the medical sequence that has been proven to lead to the best therapeutic outcomes. Consultation is often a part of initiation as well as decision-making, as cases of extreme complexity make it difficult for any one physician to have adequate insight. Many of the conflicts that face the medical team will likely evolve around smooth operation of the sophisticated technologies that the team is attempting to incorporate into patient care. Therefore, resolution of a conflict will always have an overtone of medical correctness. Compromise is not the best way of resolving a conflict related to medical care. The new systems must create an opportunity for professionals to reach consensus without wasting their time. The system must make it possible to review the medical facts, and concede a position, if indeed a mistake has been made. This learning from each other must above all be safe and supported by a common commitment to improve through positive critique rather than negative criticism. Finally, in critique and feedback, strong emphasis should be placed on scientific observations of the patient's progress after the utilization of appropriate drugs, blood, and consultation, etc. for cases that define cohort groups. The key is to focus on the best processes so that we can come to understand outcomes and how to control them.

Human Interaction

Knowing and using the best response to each others' style requires clear and direct observation in all six elements of leadership. These new skills of observation and self-awareness take the most practice and attention, because these skills have been the most neglected in our education. In the area of communication, developing a two-way dialogue that incorporates listening becomes a critical skill for the entire team, but this is only the first step in building genuine trusting human encounters necessary for high-quality care. Acquiring knowledge is no longer limited to medical technology, but also includes knowledge about the changing roles of members of the medical team, not to mention the patient's social interactions, support systems, fears, and prejudices. Gleaning this information depends on critical and more refined communication skills. When a decision is made as to medical care, communication skills and adequate knowledge about the patient ensure that this individual has true informed consent, a realistic understanding of expectations, and a sense of shared responsibility in the decision. With this foundation, the team can actually initiate the actions "with the patient." Even if the patient is hospitalized and bedridden, the emotional sense of sharing in this step is an important one.

If conflicts occur — and they are inevitable — then they need to be resolved. This requires one-on-one dialogue and is separate from the medical rightness or wrongness of care. The patient needs to ventilate anger if misunderstanding and frustration exist. The physician should never fear asking questions like, "Well, what do you think of what happened today?" even when what happened was a major medical complication. The greatest fear of the physician is that the patient will break down and cry or, worse, go into an angry tirade about how inadequate the skills of the physician are. In reality, the patient, even when angered, will focus on his or her own perceptions and fears, and give the physician a starting place to clarify the misunderstandings and the unfortunate limitations of both the technical and human aspects of medicine. By working together the team reinforces understanding.

This process of resolving conflict leads directly to critique and feedback, which offers a needed opportunity to reflect, listen, and reevaluate. The patient will appreciate the opportunity to voice opinions, positive or negative, and most will be positive. The reality is that the majority of patients, despite their pain and suffering, have an immense respect for the process of medical care. Feedback should take place with patients who have had good medical outcomes, as well as with those who have been less fortunate. Feedback not only reinforces the physician-patient relationship, but is emotionally stimulating to the entire medical team. The greatest mistake that a physician makes in providing medical care is to assume that in situations of poor-quality medical outcome the patient does not have a deep desire to discuss the steps that might have been taken differently. Being given the respect and time that this process entails often prevents a lawsuit, even when the medical decisions were in error.

Tracking Improvement

Physicians and hospital staffs are using the model presented here as a tracking tool to direct recurrent training and regularly scheduled open discussions to solidify critique and feedback, with the goal of refining the human interaction skills necessary to establish 9,9 medical teams. The physician or medical team member can pinpoint difficult patients, target the diagnoses and the difficulties in team management, and submit the data for analysis to identify process improvement in complex team interactions. An audit-type review can be made of the six elements of leadership and the impact of grid styles on the effectiveness of the medical team process can direct efforts for further improvement. This approach has proven to be invaluable as the link between CPI and case management. Collection of data and constructing a positive approach to feedback has become critical in order to constantly improve performance, morale, and outcomes to ensure that CPI makes a difference.

People Make Your Practice Work

The reality of achieving the highest quality modern medical care is that it cannot be accomplished alone. The era of one physician with a horse and buggy moving from home to home on the open frontier is long behind us. Today, the complex interactions of physician, physician extender, nurse, allied health care professional, hospital administrator, third-party payer, patient, and family support structure for the patient are inextricable.

When you ask the question, "What type of people do I want to work with as I attempt to establish 9,9 medical care?" keep your thinking basic. Ask what kind of people you think will cooperate. Find people who are optimistic, who have smiles on their faces, who believe that quality medical care is possible. A good way to determine what type of individuals you need for a supportive medical team is to ask the opposite question: "What types of individuals would totally devastate teamwork excellence?" Another way to say it is, "What characteristics of people would prevent 9,9 teamwork?" Common replies are dishonesty, narrowness, unreliability, and incompetence. If you then look for the opposite qualities in your medical team members, you will have honest individuals who are broad thinkers and are capable and reliable when it comes to task performance. The underlying fact is that the new systems of care can shape your team, even if it means letting the dead weight go. That may be hard for some organizations, but sometimes it is necessary. Keep in mind that poor team performance affects the outcome you get credit for. It is neither wise nor acceptable to accept the status quo.

After evaluating the people resource essential to your cooperative approach for excellence, recall the medical issues you have targeted and the special knowledge that your team already possesses. Next, you may realize that your success also depends on your particular location and working conditions.

Location/Accessibility

Realizing that you need a plan to achieve 9,9 medical care puts a whole new slant on where you have chosen to live and practice. Are the facilities that make up your system of care able to provide you the support that you require for excellence? What effect does your location have on your ability to be an effective participant in the new delivery models that are emerging? Can you respond to medical emergencies in a timely way? Are the technical limitations in the people you have to work with and their inability to interact effectively with others large enough barriers to your success that you would consider changing hospitals, medical groups, or even locations within the country? Is the volume of medical cases available in your particular specialty adequate to maintain the medical-technical expertise basic to 9,9 medical excellence? If the answer to any of these questions is no, then you must ask, "Do I change my medical practice to adapt to the system I have selected to support my ability to generate an income?" or "Will I risk investigating a new location that allows me to provide the type of medical care that I have defined as essential in my 9,9 medical practice?" You probably cannot answer these questions without a closer look at the next area of concern, working conditions.

Working Conditions

In considering working conditions, most of you probably think of the rules and regulations of the hospital and the operational protocols that you have established in your own offices. These can be complicated by the size of the hospital or the size of the organization in which you work. If you are in practice for yourself, then you are undoubtedly used to setting your own working conditions. If you are employed, you may have had to adjust to those already in place. The key in either event is to have made conscious choices about location, people, and the knowledge needed in the practice you have defined. These areas can be affected dramatically by the conditions under which you work.

Changing the working conditions in a new system of care can be an opportunity but it is always a bit stressful; however, the six elements of leadership can serve as a framework in this area as well. In your role as the physician leader of the team, you can easily see that care is impacted by the communication styles of those people you are working with. The way information is gathered and shared also contributes to the work atmosphere. Decisions that determine the working environment in your new system of care impact every member of your medical team, yet unilateral and authoritative decision making may have become ingrained habits. Considering the views of the experienced medical staff that make up the system can lead to working conditions that meet everyone's needs or it can lead to total chaos. Conflict resolution may be the single most important skill that shapes your working environment. If your response to conflict is to initiate critique and feedback, your team will grow and develop creative solutions to the problems that constantly emerge in the new system of care.

Carrying working conditions one step further, you may wish to look specifically at the hospitals and groups where you deliver medical care. The priority that the system has given your particular specialty will determine what equipment and facilities are available to help meet the medical-technical needs of your patients and, equally important, what commitment to staff development is made to meet the human needs of your patients. Through all of this, it is important to remember that no physician has to be a victim of circumstance. The leadership skills discussed in this book can guide you in creating working conditions that support a 9,9 medical practice in most settings. If you feel the situation is hopeless, perhaps an alternative location for your 9,9 practice exists. The hospital or clinic unable to move in this direction is unlikely to survive the demanding years ahead.

Levels of Responsibility/Budget

Separating varying levels of responsibility from their effect on income is difficult. You may find it odd not to have considered the impact of a 9,9 medical approach on your budget until this point. However, in reality, the other controlling factors have to be decided before a budget can be addressed. One of the most important influences on income will be how you approach the level of responsibility of the rest of your team.

Your role with the patient is probably either captain of the ship, leader of the team, or team member, with a say equal to that of the other members of the team. Each of these leadership styles takes different commitments of time, and time translates into money. Financial leverage comes from delegating appropriate levels of responsibility to other health care professionals who can add time and quality to the care that you are responsible for. That requires learning supervisory skills and providing clinical leadership in addition to being a good clinician. Accepting full responsibility for a perfect outcome in an imperfect world may have tremendous financial impact, as lawsuits can affect insurability, and their settlements can attach estates and future earnings. So your system, however complex, should be designed to care for all patients, even the difficult ones. What price do you put on true medical excellence? How much is it worth in the new system of care? If you can prove that your system of care is better than the system being offered by your competition, then you will get to find out the answers to these questions.

The people you select to be a part of your medical team can be chosen to maximize your contribution, but it takes new levels of responsibility for each team member. What will they earn? You must develop trust and respect not only with your patients but within this more complex medical team. For many non-medical professionals, this will mean more income. Productivity, creativity, personal satisfaction, and even health are best served when all of those participating in the care have appropriate levels of responsibility and income. Deciding how these issues will impact the real value of your care will lead to a conviction about new responsibilities that are appropriate for your medical team and whether or not you wish to be reimbursed for the added responsibility of hiring and supervising extenders of your care.

The 9,9 Approach to the Level of Responsibility

If fulfillment through contribution is the motivating force that gives the entire team its character and its support, then each individual will become committed to the success of the medical process. Team members will take responsibility for their actions, contribute significantly, and be productive and helpful to others. This is where quality becomes a reality.

Medical team members can only contribute when the information needed for creative problem solving is available to them. Because self-responsibility is key to the delivery of optimal medical care, open communication becomes essential. Shared responsibility and ultimately self-responsibility then evolve naturally.

Shared responsibility, a requirement for medical excellence, begins with the medical team. This can only be accomplished as conflicts are solved by confrontation and replaced with understanding and agreement as the basis for cooperative effort. This new understanding, in turn, creates conviction and commitment to outcomes, and outcomes improve.

9,9 Critique of Group Action

Possibly the best way to ensure that the level of responsibility will be adequate in your 9,9 medical team is through the multifaceted process of critique. The ability to use critique effectively carries tremendous power when it comes to leading others, and the step-wise process of critique can be applied to virtually every group interaction. Using critique requires conscious effort until it becomes an integral part of your team's approach to medical care.

Precritique occurs in the early phases of developing a treatment plan; team members assess past actions and create a strategy for providing optimal medical care. Concurrent critique is a process of stepping away from or interrupting an activity to study it, to assess the interactions, to consider alternatives for improving performance, and to anticipate and avoid any activities that have adverse consequences. Postcritique is a more or less natural way of reflecting on what has happened and considering suggestions for ways to improve.

When members have widespread understanding of, and are skilled in, utilizing critique, the rate at which they learn can then be accelerated. Shared responsibility in this critical step confirms that your 9,9 team will progress and accomplish the goals for high quality that you have outlined. Ongoing critique is the key to understanding responsibility and is essential in establishing and maintaining a truly excellent system of care.

Objectives, Goals, and Values

As you build your system, you will want to create the step-by-step objectives that will lead to the overall goals that have evolved from your planning. In order to work successfully together on these objectives, you and the other medical team members will need to direct your energies to attaining common goals. In the final analysis, either these goals will reflect your value system or you will have difficulty mustering the motivation to achieve them.

Personal Ownership

The concept of ownership is of primary importance. People are strongly motivated to achieve objectives when the goal belongs to them. After an individual has considered all the ramifications of reaching the goal, he or she can develop personal pride in the possibility of really reaching it. The final step is when a person gives his or her personal commitment to the challenge of attaining the goal. Once the goal has been internalized, the individual "owns" the goal and objectives are simply steps toward achievement of a desired end.

Clarity

The goal must be clear to the person responsible for reaching it. If the goal is unclear to a medical team member, that individual is unable to decide what actions he or she has to take to accomplish the goal in a meaningful way.

Meaning

Medical activities are oftentimes broken down into too many parts. The pieces by themselves may not make sense. If the goal is an arbitrary fragment of something larger, it is less likely to be a source of motivation than if it is a meaningful whole unto itself.

Significance

Even if the goal is personally owned, clear, and meaningful, it may still be perceived as unimportant. This is a typical problem created by the bureaucracy of medical care, which requires that so much paperwork become the goal of the hospital nurse. A goal is only likely to be motivating if it has apparent value. Possessing significance, then, is an important property for your goals.

Difficulty

A goal that can be accomplished with little effort lacks challenge. At the other extreme, a goal so difficult as to create a high probability of failure is also unlikely to be motivating. Sometimes a goal that appears very difficult can become inviting if its components can be dealt with as sub goals. When you are putting your overall plan together, objectives should be developed to achieve step-wise progress toward goals. The CPI process uses data to organize this effort in areas once thought too difficult to improve.

Time

An ideal goal is one that is located far enough in the future to make reaching it challenging but feasible, yet not so far away that the sense of urgency and the need to define objectives are lost. A reasonable time frame is probably 1 year in length, if it is coupled with a plan for meeting the stated objectives through the assignment of specific tasks to ensure that motivation will be sustained. Process outcomes can provide intermediate successes to keep momentum going.

Feedback

The new system of care will be of little value unless objectives can be reviewed to see if the project is moving in the direction necessary to meet the goal. The need for additional steps can be assessed. If they are needed, what is required to implement these steps can be determined. Accurate and frequent feedback on actual performance ensures the greatest progress toward meeting the goal.

Priority of Goals

Two or more goals may be established without the awareness that they are mutually incompatible. An example is two positive approaches to improving your hospital, both equally attractive: One involves long-term funding of the clinical practice improvement research and development needed to make your hospital a 9,9 facility; the other proposes launching a short-term campaign directed at improving the public image of the facility. Funds are insufficient to do both, and a splitting of funds may mean that neither is done well. The solution is establishing a "hierarchy of goals," by considering both proposals in depth. Once you understand the priority of the goal, a plan to accomplish it can be created or it will be understood to be of less urgency.

Objectives

After formulating your goal, the next step is to walk backwards from it and to identify the specific objective steps that will be necessary to realize that goal. Those engaged in the activity can test the logical progression of their proposed steps prior to finalizing them. The operational plan then becomes a working blueprint for future action. The advantage of making this step-wise evaluation is that barriers that might otherwise loom unexpectedly and insurmountably can be anticipated and dealt with in a problem-solving manner.

Making Your New Health Care Delivery System A Reality

The last step is to consider whether your current situation contains obstacles that will block the objective steps. If so, these must be resolved. To do so may require analyzing the actual situation within a hospital or clinic structure in some detail and then providing a realistic picture of priorities for the staff and the physicians.

Once priorities have been established, the activity shifts into an agreed-on "management by objectives" action program that involves supervision, consultation, and self-direction. A written plan of action can be drawn up that describes the objectives that are to be achieved. Specific steps to be taken are scheduled against time requirements, critique points are designated for the review of progress in light of the objectives, and adjustment sequences are built in to provide for unforeseen circumstances and changes in conditions. Once sound goals are in place, this "paper" program is no longer essential.

The reality is that your hospital is setting goals every day with or without you. Goals based on 9,9 excellence are no more difficult, and are far more rewarding, than those based on convention or mediocrity.

General goals that guide the steps described above can be as simple as "provide better care to patients." Byproducts of such a goal are decreased malpractice risk, a lower cost of medical care, improved self-responsibility and self-care of patients, and greater career satisfaction. If you are a mover and a shaker, and hope to motivate your entire hospital system as an alternative to leaving the area, then you are likely to demand medical excellence from facilities that have previously been unable to participate in the 9,9 process described in this book. On the other hand, you may fall into the group of physicians who want to start one step at a time in their own offices to feel out the practicality of redesigning the 9,9 medical team to assure a competitive edge.

Implementing Positive Change: Phases 1-5

The authors are dedicated to the creation of clinical practice improvement strategies that support the efforts of physicians throughout an entire community of 9,9 medical care. The first step for the self-motivated physician within this system may be to find the right person in the office or hospital to work with in creating a plan of action. Maybe your first objective will be to establish "pulse booking" appointments to keep patients from waiting or to convince your colleagues of the value of understanding 9,9 medical care. The important point is to realize the potential of this overall program and to pick an easy first objective so that you can start today. If you are looking for more structure to guide you toward your goals of ensuring the highest quality of care possible in the lowest-risk legal environment, consultation is available through PhDs, MDs, and other health care professionals who are specifically trained by Medical Resource Management in bringing programs of this nature to fruition.

Phase 1 is the self-awareness phase during which physicians, nurses, and hospital administrators complete seminars in order to clarify the issues touched upon in this book. Phase 2 focuses on the development of physician-led teamwork referred to as CPI (clinical practice improvement). In this phase, goals and objectives are tailored to the specific needs of the emerging system of care. Outmoded traditions, precedents, and past practices are replaced with a data-driven improvement in technical outcomes as well as an interdependent team culture. Personal objectivity increases during the course of medical care, because this step not only includes tracking outcomes, but it tracks team progress to evaluate interactions between all team members, including the physician and the patient. Critique is a source of learning and growth that leads to improved operational results, lower cost, higher satisfaction, and a better medical outcome. Standards of excellence are established, and objectives for team and individual achievement are clarified as steps toward mutual goals.

The third phase revolves around the resolution of conflicts between major groups such as the physicians and nurses or one specialty that works closely with another. The emphasis is on the value of conflict resolution and critique and feedback, and on overcoming the fear of conflict and enhancing the interactions between specialties and between teams that must complement each other's functions within the hospital if the highest quality care is to be the result. A series of recurrent simulation-based educational modules is introduced. A systematic framework is then used as a means of analyzing barriers to cooperation and coordination and redirecting the focus to problem-solving and decision-making skills that can be used to defuse antagonism and to resist compromise. Phase 3 is engaged in only by those groups that exhibit actual barriers to effective cooperation and coordination, and is especially important in areas where quality outcome data pinpoint a need for improvement.

In phase 4, the dynamic strategic model is expanded to meet the requirements of a truly integrated health care delivery system. The ever-changing pressures on medicine have made it clear that physicians, as part of their organizations (be they hospital or corporate), will be responsible for examining and rejecting the outmoded, unreliable, and unprofitable aspects of a health care delivery system's business logic. They will then be involved in formulating a replacement model based on the organization's definition of quality and of its future business activities in terms of a balance between the needs of society and those of the hospital, physician group, and payor. The society's need for products and services is weighed against the hospital or corporation's concern for profitability and the staff's desire for security and satisfaction in performing work that calls for participation and commitment. That language may sound odd in the field of medicine, but it directly impacts the quality of clinical medical care and it is here to stay.

Specific minimum and optimum financial objectives can be established in conjunction with a definition of the character of quality health care delivery using outcomes data, demographics information, and redesigned health care teams. The scope, nature, and depth of markets to be penetrated can be defined. A structure for organizing and integrating all aspects of the delivery of medical care can then be created, along with a plan for maintaining momentum. Policies to guide future business decision making can also be delineated in terms of the quality of clinical medical care.

Phase 4 rests on an intellectual investigation of the most basic concepts of business logic currently available. These concepts are drawn from the writings of managers who pioneered in the development of a systematic business logic, yet they are tailored to preserving the philosophies of the profession that underlie the practice of medicine. Phase 4 is completed when the evaluation of the strategic system model confirms its ability to support the delivery of optimal medical care. At that point the model is approved by the responsible executive board and by the board of directors for the integrated health care delivery system.

Phase 5 is the final implementation phase of the model developed in phase 4. With the blueprint developed in phase 4, phase 5 simply identifies and implements the objectives that must be carried out to shift from the old to the new.

Values: Some Closing Remarks

Personal Values

The motivation to achieve our personal goals lies in the values that each of us defines for ourself. In a greatly simplified form, the following three sets of values distinguish different people's attitudes about quality and about their careers:

1. Some choose to work for profit and prestige, as a way of defining themselves. The quality of the work they achieve gives them structure and meaning.

2. Others work in an attempt to grow inwardly toward self-understanding, self-realization, and inner peace, choosing to remain students of life. For them, the quality of the work they achieve demonstrates a way to grow.

3. Still others work out of a sense of commitment to society and their fellow man. These individuals find that the opportunity to give to others is reward enough to strive for quality within their work.

The chances are that you spend some time in each of these areas, but taking a moment to articulate your values leads to a fuller understanding of your motivation in life and a clearer definition of your goals and objectives and how they relate to the quality of life and work.

The goals that underlie our commitment to 9,9 medical care have evolved from our values and the shifts in values that we see across the American medical scene. It has become fundamentally clear that America cannot afford to provide unlimited access for total medical care to all of its citizens. The only solution is to give patients greater responsibility for their health. To achieve this, all individuals must have the opportunity to participate in any decision that affects their lives directly.

This is not as easy as it sounds. As we see it, three steps are necessary for this goal to be achieved:

1. The patient must believe that his or her health can indeed improve, even though medicine has its limitations. This belief makes the patient a committed member of the team. This step also emphasizes the physician's leadership role. If he or she is unable to obtain true informed consent, then a team process must be in place that will facilitate this step.

2. The individual must know what to do. The need for partnership between physicians and patients as they work together is basic if patients are to achieve high levels of self-care.

3. The most important step involves the patient's will. The patient must be able to say, "I will do it." Conviction often results from the patient's confidence in the care that is received. However, we must emphasize the personal role in self care and provide education to give patients new skills focused on sustainable versus temporary change. This step is facilitated by trust and is a place where medical care begins to impact the patient's life beyond the medical treatment, but it is more than that. The will to change rests on the patient's value system, which brings us back to your values.

To develop an understanding and common goals, you and your patients should consider the values that you share. If your values are in opposition, disaster can be the outcome of the best-laid plans. So, as esoteric as it may seem, the ethics or values that underlie your medical practice need to be discussed openly. They need to be clear to your patients, and above all else, they need to be clear to you.

Values: The Big Picture

As the field of medicine becomes increasingly affected by economic concerns, the traditional professional values of physicians are being called into question. Private practice may become a relic of history, and the survival of hospitals may rest on decisions that physicians are making daily in the course of practice.

The continuing existence of private practitioners has been challenged by the growth of large medical groups, PHOs, HMOs, and PPOs. Some observers now feel that closed panel health-management organizations represent the health care system of the future. Physicians, by active or passive participation in what is going on around them, will influence the decision-making bodies — medical societies, specialty societies, hospitals, and finally, integrated health care delivery systems — that can impact the future direction of medicine.

Hospitals, working in concert with their physicians, will resolve to use ethically based decision making in meeting the demands of quality assurance policies, utilization review boards, and the new restraints being placed on them by a government-imposed regulations and reimbursement systems, or they will abandon ethics for economics or be forced to close or turn over operations to an organization with a clear vision of the future. A strong likelihood exists that the trend of placing physicians at financial risk for the care they provide will continue over the next few years. If that continues, even greater pressure will exist for physicians to consider economics and professional ethics in medical decision-making. As physicians are forced to make painful choices with regard to rationing, the ethical grounding of medicine needs to remain clear. However, unless physicians assume a leadership role and affirm their convictions, decisions about rationing may continue to be taken out of their control. The 1988 Oregon legislation, which decreed that soft-tissue transplants could be denied to individuals on Medicaid, is but one example of economics driving medical care decision-making.

From the hospital biomedical ethics committee's point of view, if what is best for patients and the hospital cannot be weighed against the technical capacity to keep patients alive, they will continue to be sustained by sophisticated technical equipment when the quality of life is gone and expenses are no longer being reimbursed. This care meets neither the human need of the patient and the patient's family nor the need of the hospital for economic viability. A system of honest communication, joint decision making, and thorough conflict resolution is essential to prevent intensive care units as an example from literally bankrupting the system in an effort to provide the best care for patients.

To meet this challenge, hospital-based biomedical ethics committees have assumed a new significance, and the physician is key to ensuring that the decisions of these committees are based on a clear sense of ethics. These groups of people are no longer restricted to making decisions on whether or not to terminate life support for patients who are in a persistent vegetative state or who have become brain dead. They now realize they have a greater responsibility to educate physicians with regard to the realities of rationing and the impact of miscommunication and mistrust on the quality of patient care.

As a profession, medicine cannot afford to lose its ethical core. The ideals of the profession, to do no harm, to make a contribution, and to act with full integrity, form an essential foundation upon which to build the future. When 9,9 medical care becomes the norm, it will bring not only improved performance to a new level of medical excellence, but will also check against misunderstanding and unnecessary lawsuits and provide a means of coping with the economic challenges to the professional ethics of medicine. The versatility inherent in the concept of 9,9 medical excellence offers the greatest hope for maintaining the profession of medicine and conquering the challenges that lie ahead.

Notes

1. GE Cooper, MD White, JK Lauber (eds): *Resource Management on the Flight Deck.* Moffett Field, CA, National Aeronautics and Space Administration, 1980.
2. DB Feaver: Pilots learn to handle crisis-and themselves. *The Washington Post,* September 12, 1982, p. A6.
3. RN Bolles: *What Color Is Your Parachute?* Berkeley, CA, Ten Speed Press, 1988.
4. RN Bolles: *The Three Boxes of Life and How to Get Out of Them: An Introduction to Life/Work Planning.* Berkeley, CA, Ten Speed Press, 1981.

Appendix A

SELF-DECEPTION VS. THE DECEPTIVE PHYSICIAN

The Pull Toward Self-Deception

Because medicine impacts people's lives so directly, in no other profession is the temptation for self-deception as great. To continue practice, physicians need to feel that they are providing the best care possible. Otherwise, when a patient experiences a complication or simply does not respond to treatment, the physician has to bear the burden of guilt. That guilt is simply too onerous for most individuals to assume. The physician does the very best that he or she can. Yet the stresses that impact the daily life of the physician as a human being may cause the quality of performance in the six elements of leadership to vary tremendously.

How physicians justify the human tendency to be less than perfect is at the root of self-deception. The nature of the business directs the focus of rationalization to medical technique. If "the right medical-technical procedure was carried out in the prescribed manner," then guilt tends to be assuaged. This preoccupation with correct technique is understandable, considering the extreme emphasis that has been placed on medical technique from the earliest stages of medical education. The intense technical demand and fatigue that accompany medical practice lead to neglect of the human needs of physicians themselves, their colleagues, and their patients.

Self-deception is the greatest barrier to recognizing the need for change and to achieving genuine medical excellence. Prior to participating in a Caring for Difficult Patients seminar, over 70 percent of physicians perceive their medical style as 9,9. At the conclusion of an intensive seminar experience, self-perception has altered dramatically for a large number of these physicians, and they identify their dominant style as something other than 9,9. This shift indicates that although self-deception is fairly widespread, it can be overcome with the appropriate educational experience. The basic concepts of the 9,9 style as described in the six elements of leadership are not difficult. They are simply underutilized because of the pressures that physicians face in their practices on a daily basis. When physicians come to understand the basis of self-deception, it can be overcome and change then becomes self-motivated.

The Deceptive Physician

A great difference exists between self-deception (something we all fall victim to from time to time) and physicians who choose to be deceptive. These individuals, who are thought to make up a small percentage of practicing physicians, are the most difficult to reach with any sort of training and development program. They are consciously involved in a game, part of which is to escape the realities of how they actually practice. Because of this, they are very difficult to recognize, and many would prefer to believe they do not exist.

These physicians are intentionally deceptive and manipulative. They use a facade, working from behind a false front. We are all familiar with the three-story facade that hides a one-story building. It may look like a palace from the front, but the reality is that it hides a shack. This is a relatively harmless deception. No one is hurt and, once inside, the individual can assess the people and products for what they truly are, even though he or she was "lured" into a building that is not what it seemed.

The ramifications of a personal facade are something else again. Appearances, expressions, words, actions, and deeds are used to intentionally deceive the world outside. This approach to the practice of medicine can be particularly dangerous in terms of the quality of care that is delivered to the patient.

Differences Between a Grid Style and a Facade

The pure theories of the 9,1; 1,9; 9+9; 1,1; 5,5; and 9,9 orientations to physician leadership all share a basic attribute: They arise naturally from the particular set of assumptions that the physician has adopted. The behavior of the person who employs one or more of these strategies is based on the belief that this is what it means to be a physician. The consequences of actions based on this style or a combination of styles may be unexpected, but the behavior is nevertheless genuine. No counterfeit is involved.

A facade, on the other hand, is a cover for deception, intrigue, and short cuts. That sounds dramatic, but the fact is that when a facade is used, the physician is trying to achieve something that otherwise could not be assured: a high patient volume, exceptional profits, or, more recently, immunity from lawsuit. The fear of malpractice may be the single greatest stimulus that causes a physician to build a facade. The physician feels that he or she cannot allow real intentions to appear on the surface. This may even be the advice of some well-meaning defense attorney: "It's how the game is played; the key is to win" — even if the approach is manipulative and devious.

Key Motivations for Facades

A general feature of any facade is that personal thoughts and feelings are not revealed. In day-to-day interactions, the patient is given the impression that the physician is open and candid. Little or nothing in what is said or done prompts the patient to probe or question motivations, for they seem quite obvious. Yet the patient, failing to recognize the physician's true intentions, is deceived by a facade.

Two principal motivations serve as the underpinning of any facade. One is a drive for mastery and control over people. Although this is also an attribute of the 9,1-oriented physician, the goals of the two physician styles are different.

The authentic 9,1 orientation is directed to visible achievement, usually in terms of highly developed technical skills or equally well developed funds of knowledge. When involved in teamwork that goes awry, these physicians classically get sidetracked into identifying someone other than themselves as the one to blame. Their deception is not intentional, but because they desire above all else to be right, they can implicate a colleague for his or her role in a negative outcome without even realizing that their motive was to shift blame from themselves.

In contrast, the facadist's goal is private and personal. This physician derives satisfaction from controlling and influencing people and events without their knowing it. High patient volume and financial reward may be byproducts of these manipulations, but the real gratification for the facadist is covert power, in that he or she delights in "working" others as the ventriloquist pulls the strings of the dummy.

The second principal motivation of the facadist is the desire to be accepted and respected by the people with whom he or she associates. This may sound like the 5,5-oriented physician, but the intent is entirely different.

The authentic 5,5 orientation maintains the status quo and membership in select groups because these associations give pleasure. 5,5 physicians may support rules as the solution to the malpractice crisis, sometimes at the expense of their colleagues, but these physicians do not realize the negative impact of their actions on the proliferation of legal cases. They feel open and honest about their intentions.

The facade strategists, on the other hand, may feel compelled to accomplish the goals of "success" and "respect" because they are means to a personal end. They may assume a variety of styles in pursuing their goals, because facadists believe they can only accomplish their ends by masking true intentions.

The facade that is utilized may or may not be consistent over time. Depending on what the facadist believes is workable, different situations may demand a shift in tactics. The facade often has a 9,9 or a 5,5 appearance; less frequently it shows itself as 9,1; 1,9; or 1,1.

Cloaking True Intentions

A facade strategist can hide true aims in a variety of ways. One is simply to avoid getting into in-depth discussions with patients; that is, to keep conversation at a surface level. Another way of hiding is to appear passive, taking on the mantle of a 1,1-oriented physician. The difference is that the facadist takes the information provided and thinks about how it can be used. Because the physician's seeming passivity is a front, the patient is not alerted that the physician is onto something. A third approach is to direct the conversation so subtly that the patient fails to notice that the physician's opinions and attitudes are not actually being revealed. By reacting to a question with a counter query, the physician can deflect the patient's probe. A fourth way involves the physician responding to questions with a set of impressive-sounding half-truths that are phrased so as to gain favor. Still another means of cloaking true intentions is by telling an outright lie. Because the facadist's success rests on not being exposed, this physician is skilled at lying in a way that is difficult to detect.

Building and Maintaining a Reputation

The facade builder not only avoids revealing intentions, but also works hard to create a positive reputation as a cover for deceptive practices. Reputation building rests on speaking and acting consistently when in public and on having connections with everything that is generally esteemed to be "good." Through impressive social and church connections, the names, activities, and business or official functions of well-respected persons can be used to bolster personal actions. A positive reputation predisposes people to favorably interpret actions as long as none of them is startlingly at variance with the rest. If the facade emanates a quality of smoothness and polish, actual motives and ways of operating are less likely to be recognized. The appearance of integrity helps mask what really lies beneath.

Another cover-up is to express lofty convictions and socially valued ideals. Genuinely humanitarian people espouse these values and so, ostensibly, does the facade builder. Facadist behavior frequently cannot be distinguished from behavior that is motivated by valid intentions. By joining philanthropic community activities, the facadist builds a character that attracts many new patients who otherwise might have gone elsewhere. Therein lies the facadist's true motivation. When the facade builder can enlist the support of ethically grounded administrators, prominent businessmen and businesswomen, and even well-respected nurses as his or her advocates, the potential for true motives to remain hidden and for undercover personal ambitions to be furthered is greatly enhanced.

Whatever tactics are used, the intent of the facade is the same: to ensure that others perceive the physician's aims as genuine and honorable when in fact they are devious and manipulative. When patients and fellow team members perceive the facadist as a competent and caring physician, they are susceptible to the physician's influence. In this way the facadist gains personal authority, patient volume, and veneration on a scale disproportionate to actual competence and contribution.

The problem of this physician's influence on peer review is seen when seemingly out of nowhere a hospital takes punitive actions restricting privileges because a review of cases has revealed numerous situations involving poor-quality care that have been covered up. The facadist has so carefully laid a good reputation that no one can believe the injustice and those in authority bear the brunt of the criticism. Even though he or she is wise enough not to take legal actions against the hospital and risk being exposed, the facadist has succeeded in proving how unfair peer review can be, setting the stage for a successful cover-up- even when caught red handed. Quality assurance is the loser.

Motivating and Controlling Patients and the Medical Team

The facade strategist depends on expressions of approval or praise as positive ways of motivating and controlling people. The person whose self-esteem has been bolstered through compliments comes to like and admire the physician responsible for these good feelings. The assumption is that praise buys influence over patients, and hence they stay on. However, this type of physician is cunning enough to keep a close check on how each patient responds to praise, because anything that could be detected as obvious flattery might endanger credibility. By the same token, care is exercised so as not to be led astray by flattery from others.

A friendly concern, which superficially resembles the 1,9 orientation, may be read into the close attention and unqualified support given to the patient's point of view. In contrast to the 1,9 physician's genuine concern for people, the facade strategist uses people for his or her own ends. "You can catch more flies with honey than with vinegar" is a well-known adage that epitomizes the thinking of the facade strategist.

When a 9,9-oriented facade is being employed, all aspects of this Grid style may appear to be present. Data are presented objectively; the patient is helped to analyze and define requirements. Within the interview situation, consensus as to treatment may be achieved. What the physician has hidden is the perception that this patient cannot be trusted: He or she has the potential to enhance the physician's reputation and practice if appropriately impressed and to sue if disappointed. The 9,9 facade is designed to keep influential patients happy by creating the semblance of a genuine relationship.

For the physician operating behind a facade, criticism of any aspect of a patient situation, even of another physician's therapy, is ruled out. Direct critique of peers is also too risky if the objective of friendships is to exert an influence on others. By abstaining from direct confrontation, the facadist avoids the negative reactions that could ensue. However, the consequence of this subtle deception is that the person to whom these facts and opinions could have proved helpful is shortchanged.

Acting with Initiative and Perseverance

The facadist, contrary to superficial appearances, is tough minded and acts decisively when opportunity calls. People may be exploited to form alliances that are then easily and quickly set aside as the occasion demands — always with some legitimate excuse. Obstacles are seldom deterrents. If one approach does not succeed, the facadist draws back and tries another tactic until the objective is realized.

In a like manner, the facade strategist is undaunted by the difficult patient or by stresses that the patient may impose. Each situation is analyzed carefully and if the odds of success are not great, even with a "slight" bending of the hospital rules and traditional practices, then the patient is "dumped." Three physicians' names will be provided for referral, and a legitimate-sounding explanation will be given to the patient so that no questions will be asked.

Thus, in building and maintaining a personal facade, the physician 1) demonstrates a concern for people when that is advantageous, 2) uses approbation to achieve certain ends, 3) avoids direct criticism, and 4) never gives up but knows when to withdraw.

Reasons for Using Facades

The deceptive physician may actually view people as objects, setting them up for processing when that is deemed appropriate or brushing them aside when they are in the way. The facade strategy becomes the means by which these conscious manipulations can be disguised.

The facadist usually believes that personal objectives are unattainable using an open and honest approach. To the extent that power is the goal and personal pleasure comes from manipulating others, the physician who employs a facade may believe that it is the only effective means for gaining these ends. This conviction is as potent in governing personal behavior as any of the assumptions that underlie the various Grid styles.

Another reason for establishing and maintaining a facade is that some physicians, for whatever reason, do not value mutual trust between themselves and patients. They are forced to create an impression that candor, helpfulness, and honesty are central to their medical approach in order to achieve their personal goals more easily. The physician who uses a facade is not governed by commonly accepted standards for maintaining social morality, let alone professional ethics. The impact on the quality of care is easy to imagine.

The tragic aspect of the medical practice that has become a facade is that if the underlying assumptions were different, if the facadist believed that a satisfying practice could be achieved and personal ambitions fulfilled through medical care with integrity, the energy and resourcefulness needed to maintain the facade could be directed to that end rather than to deception. Admittedly, some facade strategists get a distorted thrill out of "living dangerously" and achieving by complex maneuvers what could have been reached by a direct approach. Most of the physicians who have adopted deceptive practice strategies simply lack sufficient confidence in their own abilities to address the responsibilities of medicine head on. In medicine, the approach used by the facadist is thought to be rare.

Summary

Behavior that results from self-deception is manifested when the underlying motivation is unknown, even to the physician. Not only are others deceived, but the physician is also a victim of this deception. Psychiatry and clinical psychology have described these tricks of the mind that allow personal motivations to be unclear and that preclude their being identified or described to others. If directly confronted with the possibility of self-deception, the individual denies it. To complicate matters further, the behavior observed always contains components of the theories under which the physicians believe they are operating.

Self-deception is a phenomenon that impacts every individual's life. It is in some way linked to fear — fear of failure, fear of the burden of guilt, fear of an uncertain future. In our seminars physicians perceive the 9,9 style as the most fulfilling and "best" way to practice. Because of self-deception (sometimes called rationalization), individuals perceive other practice styles (9+9; 9,1; 5,5; 1,9; and even 1,1) as 9,9. This is usually because they perceive 9,9 qualities as ideal and they intend to be 9,9. Intention overshadows the actions that are observed. The difference between the theory and the reality of medical practice is that for various reasons physicians are not aware when they slip away from the 9,9 style. Any physician who assumes that he or she is always 9,9 is a victim of self-deception. This book and the educational programs for which it provides the theoretical underpinnings are dedicated to building skills of self-perception, developing an understanding of patient styles, and establishing the basis for effective interactions with medical team members. Good, clear observation of one's self and others is free of self-deception. The ability to eliminate self-deception is also the subject of much writing about truth, peak performance, enlightenment, success, and even God and church.

At the other end of the scale, the physician consciously constructs a facade to mask the pursuit of personal and private goals. Insofar as observable behavior goes, this physician appears well intentioned and true motivation is hidden. The individual is likely to be seen as practicing in one of the styles described in previous chapters. Because tactics vary in order to take advantage of opportune situations and people's weaknesses, the facade strategist may be difficult to identify unless the physician's activities are tracked over a period of time. The use of facades to cloak intentions constitutes a personal barrier for any physician to achieve 9,9-oriented relationships with both patients and associates.

Facade strategists can be highly successful, but they are a potential Achilles' heel to all members of the medical team and to medicine in general. The lack of integrity inherent in a facade means that medicine is being represented to patients by a physician undeserving of trust. The resultant behavior is likely to lead to genuine injury that can have a tremendous boomerang effect when patients and lawyers eventually discover that the facadist has been manipulating situations for personal gain. This physician is the individual who has done the most to discredit physicians and to tarnish the reputation of medicine as a valuable caring profession.

Appendix B

RED FLAGS, OR "I THOUGHT I WAS 9,9 BUT..."

Identifying your dominant Grid styles is a crucial first step in the process of ensuring a professional career of constant growth and improvement-becoming more 9,9. The next step is beginning to recognize those ingrained habits that reinforce behaviors that you may be trying to change. Once you have created the environment for an effective system of critique and feedback, members of your team can use the following red flags as keys to aspects of your behavior that reflect Grid styles other than 9,9. As you develop this system of support, it may be helpful to occasionally review the red flags inherent in the various Grid styles. The 9,9 alternatives present ways of interacting with your patients and the other members of your team that represent concrete steps toward the delivery of truly excellent medical care.

"Of Course, I'm Really 9,9, But What if I Lean Toward A 9,1-Oriented Practice?"

Communication

One-Way Communication. The goal of 9,9 communication is to create a two-way exchange. If you feel defensive when others have something to communicate, that may be a sign of "one-way listening." The best approach when this happens is to stop, take a deep breath, fight off any anger, and analyze what the patients, or your peers for that matter, are trying to communicate to you. Trust is built through understanding, not through overwhelming people with information or your authority.

Anger. If anger persists, that is a real red flag. The biggest challenge in communication for the 9,1-oriented physician is to control emotions, anger most specifically. In order to understand the source of your anger, you might ask, "Why am I angry?" Then take a deep breath, wait for an answer, and use your conclusion to resolve the anger that you are feeling.

Yes/No Questioning. If all you ever hear in response to your questions are yes or no answers, that may be a problem. The involvement of others can be promoted by getting them to say what they think before you state your position. Otherwise, the strength of your convictions may eliminate their participation altogether. Try the questions, "What are your thoughts on how we can solve your problem?" or "What questions do you have?"

Unrealistic Patient Expectations. The one-way listening flag mentioned above may be the cause of unrealistic expectations. A genuine sense of realistic expectations involves more than agreeing to therapy; realistic expectations exist when the patient is aware of the limitations of medical expertise, and *trusts* and understands you and your advice. Analyzing your own expectations for perfection and your assumptions about the patient's role in your care is a critical step in achieving realistic expectations.

Acquiring Knowledge

Dull Patients. A 9,1 flag may be raised if you find yourself discounting information because you lack respect for a patient's intelligence. The physician's assessment of the patient's need for medical care is critical, but medical needs can be put into perspective with the patient's perceived need. Although patients rarely have an adequate supply of medical knowledge to make decisions unilaterally, they are experts on themselves and their own perspectives. They are very clear about the impact of their illness on their job, family, sense of identity, sexuality, and ability to return to what they consider a normal lifestyle. This information can have a major impact as you weigh alternative treatment plans.

Avoiding Consultation. One of the major difficulties for the 9,1-oriented physician is overcoming the pride that prevents him or her from consulting individuals who have information that might improve the quality of care. This tendency to avoid consultation is widespread, as evidenced by the fact that many hospitals have had to institute rules and regulations that require consultation. Accepting the fact that no one can expect to be the absolute expert on every aspect of medicine is a step toward medical excellence.

Decision Making

Quick Decisions. The ability to arrive at decisions quickly can be a red flag. Explaining why you are ignoring the advice of others can be more than "because I know more than they do." Communicating the rationale behind your decision, rather than stating the conclusion only, is an excellent way to educate both staff and patients and moves you into the area of true communication. It also provides a check for you, as you may find times when you cannot explain the rationale for your decision. Logic then dictates that you go back, review the literature, reconsider the individual situation, and verify your conclusion.

Patients Who Do Not Share in the Responsibility for the Outcome. If you have the tendency to dominate patients, you may be taking full responsibility for perfect outcomes. Because some patients may wish to abandon responsibility in the health care process, this is a red flag that you must constantly be on the alert for. Drawing patients into the decision-making process leads to joint decision making and a sense of shared responsibility for the outcome.

Initiative

Calling All of the Shots. If patients or the members of your medical team are responding as if their only options are to salute you or stay out of your way, you have identified another red flag. Rather than immediately bursting in to solve the problem when an emergency arises, take a moment to observe your team. You may see that they are not responding to obvious needs, possibly because they are waiting for you to tell them what to do. You may need to shift away from the captain of the ship in order to become the leader of high-quality teamwork.

Conflict Resolution

Liking a Good Fight. Conflict is inevitable; but anger, the 9,1 response, is inappropriate in medical care and signals the need for change. Ignoring this response to conflict and accepting anger as part of a colorful personality are common reactions. The step that follows is to blame others when the aftermath of conflict is less than favorable. Finally, an excuse or rationalization will be used to eradicate personal responsibility for the whole situation.

Patients Who Just Won't Listen. Patient objections are common, and the temptation to overwhelm the objection with information is almost second nature due to traditional medical education. Your job, as hard as it may be with difficult patients, is to present the needed information in an understandable form and be sure the patient hears it. Patient objections may be a sign that you have not succeeded. More patience may be the solution.

Critique and Feedback

Depending on Informed Consent Contracts. If you think that informed consent is a contract, or only applies to surgical approaches, that is a red flag. Rather than asking a patient to sign on the dotted line, you can ask, "How will you cope with complications if they occur?" You can wait for the answer, or you can push for a signature on a contract. The latter is a barrier to trust and to medical excellence.

"Of Course, I'm Really 9,9, But What if I Lean Toward A 1,9-Oriented Practice?"

Communication

Not Discussing Medical Issues. If you have to remind yourself that you should be addressing the medical issues and then ignore the reminder because you are enjoying the friendly conversation so much, you can ask yourself, "Why don't I feel comfortable discussing the technical aspects of the situation with the patient?" Either you or the patient or both of you prefer other topics, and you are an expert at meeting human needs. Nevertheless, coming to an understanding of the technical issues is essential to the delivery of high-quality care.

Unrealistic Patient Expectations. Patients depend on your friendly and caring attitude, but they also expect the very best and latest in medical expertise. Your desire to be liked and to be popular is in the balance with the patient's expectation for the high-quality medical care required in this highly technical era. By modifying medical advice to meet what you perceive as the emotional needs of the patient, you may be misinterpreting the patient's expectation. Patients may prefer not to discuss the treatment plan, but that does not negate their expectation for the best medical outcome. Establishing realistic expectations about the outcome in technical *and* emotional terms eliminates the potential for surprise.

Acquiring Knowledge

Hating Continuing Medical Education Courses. Not liking to read medical journals or attend lectures is a particular problem for the 1,9 physician. Although the current state of continuing medical education (CME) may be part of the problem, it cannot be used as an excuse. The continual advances in medicine demand that the physician read and study in order to provide the best medical care. Identifying journal articles that are relevant to your practice and setting aside some time each day to read them might be a way to begin.

Shunning Consultation. To avoid exposing ignorance, the 1,9 physician shies away from consultation. Yet a common-sense way of strengthening medical expertise is to ask experts questions that invite explanations. Knowledgeable consultants are generally willing to contribute what they know and will respect your interest in them as experts at the same time that they provide a high-quality and free education. You are already an expert at gathering information from patients; moving that enthusiasm toward acquiring technical knowledge from fellow physicians can be a major step toward excellence.

Decision Making

Feeling Sorry for Patients. Hesitating to reach a decision because you feel compassion for the patient is misdirected concern. Embarrassing or unpleasant decisions are unavoidable in medical practice, and postponing the decision only delays the inevitable.

Patients Making the Wrong Decision. The patient does not have the resources necessary to make a medical decision alone. When you are tempted to let the patient make the decision, see that as a red flag. Shared responsibility is important, but the burden of decision is never fairly placed on the shoulders of the patient.

Changing Your Mind. If a medically sound decision has been made, yet the patient is unhappy about it, the reasoning behind the medical decision needs to be explained in greater detail. Shifting from a majority opinion to a minority opinion that you usually do not use may be an indication that you are succumbing to the pressure of a difficult patient. If you feel insecure about your position, you might want to turn to a colleague for advice.

Initiative

Asking for the Patient's Permission to Act. Once a sound decision about therapy has been made and action is needed, waiting for the patient's okay brings your decision into question. Rather than asking for the seal of approval from a patient who lacks the medical background to make the decision, you can ask the patient to participate in carrying out the plan.

Taking a Back Seat to Your Colleagues. If it has been years since you volunteered to do a grand rounds or a nursing in-service, you are likely to feel ill prepared. Volunteering to speak on a topic that interests you will provide motivation to become the expert once more.

Conflict Resolution

Doing Anything to Avoid a Fight. Conflict is inevitable, no matter how great your social skills, so be conscious of how often you abandon the battlefield. Differences can be examined without creating tension, risking personal rejection, or going to war. Initially, resolution may be more work than running away and, depending on the style of the person you face, may make you uncomfortable, but it is a critical step to medical excellence.

Going Along with Others Even Though You Were Right. If others disagree with you, notice how often you immediately adopt their point of view. Before you surrender, restate your position and ask them to explain their reservations. Make a conscious decision as to whether you believe they are right or wrong, and move forward with conviction. If some doubt remains in your mind, seek out a third opinion.

Feeling Guilty When Patients Are Upset. Objections should not be taken as a personal insult. They usually reflect disenchantment or disappointment with regard to expectations or medical outcome, especially in light of a physician who is so good at meeting psychological and emotional needs. By discussing the objections, you can usually come to mutual understanding that eliminates the patient's concerns.

Critique and Feedback

Feeling Guilty When There Is a Bad Outcome. Your orientation is naturally supportive and sincere, but when empathy regarding a poor outcome turns to guilt it is always a red flag. Looking for barriers to good performance, both within yourself and in the medical team providing care to your patients, is essential to high-quality medical care. Future problems can be prevented by correcting negative situations, but feelings of guilt do little or nothing to improve the outcome. Focus on positive steps that can be taken, rather than dwelling on the past.

What They Signed for Is Not What You Did. Because patients do not have enough information when you allow them to make medical decisions, objections that result in your changing the original therapy also alter the information needed for true informed consent. Informed consent cannot be assumed; you need to bring the patients to an equally high level of understanding of the alternative therapy. If you explained to them that you deferred to their wishes for the purpose of meeting their human needs, they may not believe the decision they made is medically sound, even though they requested or approved the procedure. Ensuring that the document they sign reflects the therapy you will provide is a means of clarifying that you and your patient have a mutual understanding of the plan for care.

"Of Course, I'm Really 9,9, But What if I Lean Toward A 9+9-Oriented Practice?"

Communication

Trying to Get Patients to Agree. Getting patients to understand is important, but if you believe that the purpose of a physician-patient exchange is to convince the patient that your way is the "only" way, that is a red flag. The compassion and dedication you feel make it very difficult to see that this style of medical practice has limitations. From the patient's point of view, the primary shortcoming is that communication is totally controlled by the physician, and the result is that realistic expectations are never achieved. Instead of being so intent on convincing the patient, you may wish to try active listening, believing that he or she has something of value to contribute.

Feeling Like a Parent. If you have the sense of a parent talking to a child who is incompetent to do anything other than listen and obey, then you might want to honestly assess your patient. Determine the level on which you can have a relationship as two adults, and develop two-way communication that meets all of the patient's needs.

Patients Who Want to Be Taken Care Of. A dependent relationship in which patients want to get well but also want you to take responsibility for their care is a red flag. Although this relationship meets the need of the 9+9 physician to take care of patients, it creates expectations of perfection that cannot always be fulfilled. The physician needs to share the limits of the treatment with the patient in order to establish realistic expectations — even if this goes against the natural inclination of both the physician and the patient.

Placing High Value on Loyalty. Loyalty, the hallmark of a paternalistic patient-physician relationship, is in itself a red flag. Unfortunately, the close emotional bond that strong loyalty engenders can be volatile, as disappointed love can move quickly to hate. The only way around this one is to develop a partnership and to establish shared responsibility.

Acquiring Knowledge

Being Driven. If you have an overwhelming sense of dedication and almost moralistic zeal about the role of the physician, if you feel like an omnipotent decision maker literally responsible for the life and death of those who come to you with grave illness, if you are a perfectionist who preaches about the virtues of medical care delivered in the only "right" way, those qualities represent another red flag. Their impact on your approach to acquiring knowledge is also significant. It takes a good listener to realize that the individual with whom you interact is also in the process of acquiring knowledge. Many adults have very well-formed ideas about what they will or will not accept in the way of advice from a physician. Overwhelming them with your convictions about the best medical approach may not provide them the opportunity to learn about you or to fully understand the impact that the treatment plan you are proposing will have on their lives. The temptation of the 9+9 physician is to acquire knowledge from all sources except the patient. Adding that store of information will add a new dimension to the care you provide.

Listening as a Technique to Get the Patient to Agree. The knowledge base that physicians acquire has always been highly medically-technically oriented. This introduces a prejudice about the value of listening to patients and attempting to meet their emotional and personal needs. If the only information you want from patients is the reassurance that you have convinced them, no matter how long that takes, you cannot form a partnership based on mutual understanding. Listening can lead to a knowledge base upon which the best decision can be determined.

Decision Making

Believing that Hospitals Do Not Need to Change. If you are comfortable with the environment that exists in the vast majority of hospitals in this country and believe that physicians should be doing the thinking for the medical team members, specifically the nurses who carry out their orders, that is a red flag. The result is team members who know what is expected of them, but who are paralyzed from making any decisions on their own. As medicine becomes increasingly complex, the physician who assumes total responsibility becomes ever more vulnerable. Involving team members in joint decision making leads to shared responsibility and a team that is not dependent on you for direction at every step along the way.

Making Decisions Unilaterally. To dominate even the childlike patient and to assume full responsibility for a perfect outcome constitute a major red flag. No matter what limitations the patient may have, some role can be defined that will help him or her become more involved in decisions about care. By determining the styles of your patients, you can plan strategies to build shared goals and mutual responsibility.

Feeling that the Medical Team Is Limited to You and the Patient. If you are involving the patient but no other team members in decisions, your concept of team may be too narrow. Sitting down with the entire medical team to hear their ideas and consider alternatives before reaching a decision is a 9,9 approach.

Initiative

Hospital or Office Staff Standing at Attention. If your medical team has been well indoctrinated and they stand at attention and wait for orders when initiative is needed, a red flag should flash in your mind. When medical team members are left powerless and ill equipped to initiate actions on their own, devastating slowdowns and possibly life-threatening inefficiencies can result. Your task may be to encourage independent thinking, feedback, ongoing education, and full utilization of the resources necessary to create the leadership abilities that will free you, the team leader, to think clearly and move ever closer to medical excellence.

Cross-Checking to Be Sure Orders Are Being Followed. If your approach to your team, no matter how well intended, is a series of cross-checks to be sure that patients and medical personnel alike are simply following orders, this is another red flag. The appropriate question to ask is, "What is the role of each individual, and how can his or her unique skills contribute to high-quality teamwork?" If an alternative plan of action is suggested, do you evaluate it for soundness prior to vetoing it? If you realize that your assumption is that your team members are only capable of carrying out orders, you can change. It is a matter of style and of believing that team members have skills that you have previously discounted.

Conflict Resolution

Using Praise and Reprimand to Avoid Conflict. Your tendency may be to avoid conflict by delivering a series of compliments and reprimands to both patients and medical team members. To ensure that you are beyond criticism yourself, you may strive for the loyalty and respect of your team. When you find yourself avoiding conflicts in these ways, try to understand the origin of the conflict in the first place, as its resolution will prevent antagonism and a replay of this situation in the future.

Disowning Patients When They Have Offended You. It is a red flag to "disown" a patient, no matter how insulting he or she has been during the interaction. Instead, given the right opportunity, the patient may be willing to explain the source of his or her anger. Once the anger is ventilated, the patient may decide to go elsewhere, or you may feel that a communication barrier between the two of you indicates that his or her needs may be better met by another physician.

These two solutions to conflict are preferable alternatives to punishing the patient by depriving him or her of the excellent care that you can provide. Resolving the issues that angered the patient may, in fact, allow you to establish a genuine relationship with the patient.

Feeling Betrayed by Patients. If you find yourself with a knot in your stomach and a sense of betrayal as you deal with an unhappy patient, this too is a red flag. Patients who object are trying to provide you with invaluable information about their perceived need, if not their real need. By constructively dealing with their complaints through open-ended questions and attentive listening, and by not taking their criticisms "personally," a higher level of patient responsibility can be achieved.

Critique and Feedback

Feedback Is Required to Keep People in Line. If you think constant feedback is necessary to ensure that the patient and medical team members are complying with the dictums you have made, then, even though you are compulsive about obtaining feedback, you are missing the opportunity to learn in the process. That is a red flag. As the leader of the team, feedback can be invaluable. Open communication and critique that involve all team members are necessary to evaluate issues such as the coordination of effort, sequential decision making, ongoing inquiry, and shifts in initiative necessary to keep the medical plan dynamic. Limiting your sources of information through a subconscious belief that all of the important knowledge has been obtained through medical education and past experience, and that your team members cannot contribute to that knowledge base, is a major barrier for the 9+9 physician. Listening to others, especially when more than one person shares the same feedback about your actions (not your intentions), is a valuable source of realistic reappraisal, moving you ever closer to medical excellence.

Being a Mentor. One type of feedback that makes the process of changing from the 9+9 orientation particularly difficult is that used in the mentor-protégé relationship. The hallmark of medical education has been to use the experience and wisdom of a senior physician as one basis for strengthening the leadership skills of physicians in training. The mentor-protégé model is actually a red flag, as it is classically 9+9 and assumes that the only feedback of value is provided by the mentor. Dependency is expected and produced in the protégé.

Realizing the pitfalls in the mentor-protégé model can help you see that even this time-honored traditional system of education and feedback can be improved. The most important factor in ensuring the validity of the mentor-protégé model is that the mentor is not a classic 9+9 physician satisfying personal needs for adulation and that the protégé uses the leadership skills acquired from the mentor to enhance the overall working of the medical team. If you have been elevated to the mentor role, that is a red flag. You are in a powerful position and may need to be alert to the temptations described here. You can deliberately choose to move toward open learning and discussion, from which you can gain as much as you give.

Expecting "Good" Patients to Be Respectful and Obedient. Failure to reach an understanding of the reason for patient compliance prior to delivering medical care is not only a red flag, but it has brought this physician style to the forefront in courtrooms. As you develop genuine partnerships with your patients, you can become alert to whether the patient is simply obeying an order to meet the expectations you have created as a 9+9 physician or whether that patient genuinely understands not only the medical care, but also his or her role in carrying out the medical plan. Realizing that a "good" patient may not be synonymous with a passively compliant one is a step towards 9,9 medical care.

"Of Course, I'm Really 9,9, But What if I Lean Toward A 1,1-Oriented Practice?"

The 1,1-oriented retreat occurs when no other action is sufficient to overcome the obstacles or barriers that face physicians. The reason 1,1 red flags are so difficult to recognize in yourself is that remnants of your dominant Grid style from the "good old days" still survive. You may continue to communicate as you did in the past, use the same medical-technical language, keep the same hours, and dress in the appropriate unwritten code of the physician. Maintaining a subdued interest in daily events, smiling or nodding acceptance, keeps the outside world from seeing a change that you yourself may not want to admit. However, deep inside you know that something is different, and that is where the red flags are helpful.

Personal Attitudes that Constitute Red Flags

Feeling Medicine Has Let You Down. Discouragement takes its toll along the road of medical care when you strive with all your heart for excellence and then are faced with the inevitable, if infrequent, failures of "the miracle of medicine." A sense of failure and subsequent discouragement constitute a red flag. Once the vicious cycle of pessimism is established, each new failure reinforces the attitude of "Why try?" Instead, you need to work with your team to assess the reasons for poor outcomes, develop a plan for change, and then initiate the steps to bring it to fruition. Once that cycle is broken, you will recover the resilience needed to accept that medicine does not guarantee perfection.

Self-Alienation. Self-alienation is another red flag. If you were once motivated by high ideals and are now letting economics dictate the decision to treat a given condition with a high-paying procedure rather than the conservative approach, your self-esteem may erode as you begin to rationalize, "It's just not worth it to continue the game." You may start to withdraw both mentally and emotionally, until a 1,1 "get by" approach becomes a dominant orientation. Reevaluating your business decisions and the extent to which you are willing to let them affect medical care may be the first step back to the profession of medicine.

Feeling You Have Practiced Too Long. A certain pull toward the 1,1 orientation is something most physicians experience if they practice long enough. Energy resources can diminish as a person advances in years, and the result may be a 1,1 orientation to medicine. Although this response may be primarily an age-related factor, other circumstances can bring this reaction at any age. An analysis of why you continue to practice may provide the motivation either to change or to leave the field of medicine.

When You Get Tired, Feeling Like It's OK to be 1,1. Sleep deprivation and fatigue are common rationalizations for 1,1 behavior, but they do not alter the reality of your situation or the outcome. When you become aware of having slipped into the 1,1 corner, this "red flag" in itself may be sufficient to cause you to bounce out and to regain energy and involvement.

Feeling the Challenge of Medicine is Gone. Burnout is a red flag that results when the rewards of work diminish over time. Much of medicine may seem routine and boring, so that a hollowness sets in and nothing seems able to replace what once may have been meaningful and satisfying work. The recommended medical treatment for burnout may be rest, relaxation, and a change of pace, but these are only temporary diversions. The real cure may be to find new challenges and interests, either within or outside the field of medicine.

Depression, Anxiety, or Taking Drugs. If you have slipped into the 1,1 corner or have gotten there via burnout and now know that is where you are, such a self-diagnosis is certainly disconcerting. If this negative motivation for change leaves you feeling depressed, being anxious, or turning to drugs, then professional help can be critical in the process of taking the necessary steps back to a more rewarding life.

Communication

The Feeling that You Can't Get Involved. If the patient-physician interaction has become tedious and rote, that is a red flag. The likelihood is great that no genuine communication is taking place between you and your patients. Try to open up and develop a human interaction. Sometimes taking a different approach is a means of restoring enthusiasm, and the impact of enthusiasm on communication is great.

Acquiring Knowledge

Finding Journals and Continuing Medical Education a Waste of Time. If your response to medical journals that come across your desk is to throw them in the trash can, almost out of habit because it has been so long since you have even thumbed through the table of contents, that is a red flag. Selecting CME courses on the basis of location rather than subject matter might also be a clue.

Listening when other physicians discuss advances and hearing peers review cases other than your own are excellent ways to gain continuing medical education. In addition, specialty organizations and the American Medical Association have developed continuing medical education tapes that can be listened to on an automobile tape player while driving to and from work. These common-sense summaries of recent advances are generally oriented toward application in the real world of medical practice. Armed with what you have just heard on a tape, it is easy to enter into a conversation and discuss what you "know" about the latest advance. Approaching the conversation from a higher-than-average knowledge base reinforces the information and demonstrates to others that you are actively gathering new knowledge in your field.

Not Caring if Difficult Patients' Needs Are Being Met. When a difficult patient seems unhappy with a diagnosis or discontent with the original recommendation for treatment, you may find yourself giving up, rather than gathering the additional information needed to answer the patient's concerns. If this red flag is ignored, patient objections may escalate into a lawsuit. Taking the extra time to uncover the real source of the patient's negative feelings is a concrete step toward 9,9 medical care.

Decision Making

Not Wanting to Lead the Team. You may feel uncomfortable at the thought of assuming command of your medical team, and the team may appear skeptical of this dramatic change in your behavior. In situations that make you feel secure, try taking a clear stand. You may be surprised by the positive response from the medical team if you have forgotten how it feels to be the leader. This new attitude provides the motivation to acquire enough knowledge to be the decision maker we have come to associate with the physician-led medical team.

Walking Away from Patients You Find Frustrating and Unrewarding. Your tendency may be to let the patient make the decision about care with only minimal guidance from you. This gulf between physician and patient makes the practice of medicine less rewarding and perpetuates the 1,1 orientation. It is easy to be uninvolved if the decision is not your responsibility.

You may find some patients more difficult than others, but their attitudes should not preclude them from the opportunity to receive care. Identifying a reasonable role for each patient clarifies the level of responsibility that he or she is expected to assume. Shared responsibility can also protect you if a poor outcome occurs. Establishment of this sort of responsibility is a major step toward moving out of the 1,1 corner.

Initiative

Not Having the Will to Initiate an Action. If you find yourself paralyzed when a situation demands an active response, this is a red flag. You have undoubtedly acted decisively in the past, so your inability to act needs to be assessed. If fear of failure is the barrier, what is the source of that fear? How can it be alleviated? If motivation is the key, then it is more a matter of will than skill, and it is the will you need to bolster.

Conflict Resolution

Walking out Mentally When Faced with Disagreement. Disappearing mentally when nurses and patients disagree with you is a red flag. The alternative is to explore and resolve the differences. Team members and patients may be disagreeing because you have not stated your case clearly. If you make your convictions known so that patients and nurses understand your position, they can react accordingly. You can stimulate feedback as a means of pooling all available resources in the quest for a solution. When the team works together to resolve conflict and to arrive at the best decision, the sense of camaraderie is energizing.

Ignoring Patient Objections. Objections are rarely a statement of "I don't want medical treatment" or a direct criticism of the care you have provided. Instead of reacting as if the objections are a personal affront, work to uncover the source of the objections and to restate the needed information in a more understandable form. Focusing on both the medical-technical and personal needs of the patient may provide the necessary perspective to work for genuine medical excellence.

Critique and Feedback

Avoiding Feedback. If you receive no feedback, you may wish to consider whether you have instilled this behavior in those with whom you work. No criticism at all may reflect that the staff does not care that they have also fallen into 1,1 behavior in the area of critique and feedback, or that they feel feedback is unwelcome. Positive, constructive criticism provides insights about the way your team members see your role as physician coordinator. Concrete suggestions may be just what you need to begin to change.

Not Taking the Time to Reach Informed Consent. The idea that informed consent is getting the patient to sign on the dotted line, therefore absolving the physician and hospital from any responsibility for poor outcome, can be a 1,1 red flag. When the nurse places a contract in your hand and requests that you "get the patient to sign this," you can stop and ask yourself what information the patient must have in order to understand the care you are about to deliver. This sounds simple, but by stopping and asking this question and then taking the five or ten extra minutes for two-way discussion regarding the procedure or treatment being recommended, you can create true informed consent. If the patient does not understand because of his or her educational level or the emotional overtones carried by the diagnosis, then he or she is risky for you to care for. With less than an optimal outcome, this patient will be unhappy. If the emergency is not life threatening, you may even feel that it is appropriate to put the patient on hold, stating that he or she may not be ready for the treatment. This response is not resignation, because your plan includes rescheduling an appointment with the patient, sitting down, and going through a more thorough process to achieve true informed consent. Once consent is obtained, along with the signature, the patient is ready to proceed; and you have taken a major step toward medical excellence.

"Of Course, I'm Really 9,9, But What if I Lean Toward A 5,5-Oriented Practice?"

Communication

Shifting Your Style to Achieve Agreement. Feeling that you need to assume a different style in response to patients of varying styles is a red flag. Although you may be tempted to accommodate the patient in any way that you can, a consistent 9,9 approach is a safer and more satisfying alternative. Playing the chameleon in an attempt to maneuver patients in a planned direction can have unforeseen results, particularly in the case of a less-than-perfect outcome. Gaining acceptance of care is not the same as gaining understanding. Winning the patient over by appearing to meet his or her needs lays a weak foundation upon which to build genuine communication and trust.

Pushing Patients Toward Acceptance of Care. When you feel yourself spurring the patient on toward a decision because you believe it is correct, this red flag indicates that you may be reacting to a resistance on the part of the patient, probably due to a lack of sound knowledge. Rather than pressuring the patient into a decision through well-practiced techniques with which you are comfortable, you can invite the patient to question your therapy. If problems surface, the dialogue can be continued until the patient has a clear expectation regarding the limitations of the medical care.

Acquiring Knowledge

Asking Questions with the Intention of Plugging Patients into a Diagnosis. Asking a prescribed set of questions in order to categorize patients so that they can be managed in a routine manner is a red flag. If you sound like you are running through a check-off list, the patient may become skeptical about your approach. Even if the symptoms immediately suggest a diagnosis, in-depth questioning may uncover something less obvious. You can accept that some subtle variation in care may be called for because virtually every patient has unique needs.

Feeling that Patients' Needs Fall into a Small Number of Categories. If all your patients' needs fit into a limited number of neatly prescribed treatments and the writing of prescriptions and rendering of advice have become routine and restricted in scope, you might ask yourself why medicine is no longer complex. Have you intentionally restricted your practice, or have you stopped considering all the options? Listening and questioning are keys to developing the knowledge base that will equip you to meet the special needs of all of your patients.

Decision Making

Going Along with the Crowd. Using the expressions *That's the way everybody else does it* or *We've always done it that way* as the reason for your decision is a red flag. When you hear yourself using statements like these to justify a decision, look for a basis in concrete facts. You can let others know the alternative possibilities that you are considering. If someone has a different plan or minority opinions have been expressed, you can evaluate them carefully and then explain the reasons you have rejected them in making your final decision. This procedure will motivate you to actively consider alternatives and to take renewed interest in decisions.

Agreeing to Disagree. When a decision involves teamwork, compromise and shading of differences constitute a red flag. In order to be sure that you are taking full advantage of the knowledge and experience of the members of your team, you can concentrate more attention on the sources of agreement and the reasons for reservations and doubts. Once your team comes to realize that compromise is no longer the desired outcome, decisions will result from clear resolution of the alternatives. The ultimate decision may be one of the original suggestions or a creative outgrowth of a number of ideas.

The Status Quo or Using Rules Instead of Thinking. Discounting the idea that others are interested in knowing what you really think, not necessarily what the rules and regulations state, is a red flag. Policies, although devised to help solve dilemmas, should not dictate your convictions. By expressing your ideas and the basis for your decision, you will encourage open communication and greater efficiency in those with whom you work.

Guiding Patients in a Preset Direction. If a smooth-running office and efficient movement of patients are your ultimate goals, you may be unable to define an appropriate level of responsibility for each of your patients. Shared responsibility for an outcome demands two-way communication, and that cannot be achieved by a cookbook procedure in a prescribed length of time. If you actively guide the participation and involvement of your patients because of time pressures, you may be assuming the responsibility for a perfect outcome. A preferable alternative might be to provide them with information, discuss why the therapy is tailored to their individual needs, and obtain a commitment on the part of the patients to participate in the care that you prescribe.

Initiative

Hanging Onto the Past. Overreliance on traditions, precedents, or past practices can have a negative impact on your ability to act in the best interests of the patient. This is not to say that you should follow unproven practices, but simply that care can be individualized on the basis of the situation that you face. If you have a clear sense of the problem and how best to solve it for a particular patient, you can move ahead with authority and generate the respect of the patient and other team members as well. The tradition of medicine is important, but action directed to meeting the unique needs of patients remains the key.

Conflict Resolution

Emphasizing the Positive. Avoiding objections by emphasizing the positive features of a treatment and ignoring the patient's or team member's original complaint altogether is a red flag. Whether they originate from a patient or another team member, you can assume that objections are at least partially justified. Rather than trying to smooth over the conflict and keep everyone happy, explore the concerns that are voiced as an opportunity to resolve differences and come to a clearer understanding of mutual goals. Conflict can be creative and constructive; it need not be seen as something destructive and to be avoided at all costs.

Critique and Feedback

Avoiding Feedback Because It Wastes Time. If your attitude reflects your belief that feedback is, at best, a waste of time and, at worst, counterproductive, you are not likely to receive much. Assuming that feedback has few (if any) redeeming qualities is a red flag. You can actively seek out feedback or you can avoid it. Indicating to people that you genuinely want feedback and critique is likely to encourage your co-workers to solve real concerns that hamper their own productivity, and it can ultimately save time. Assumptions that you have made about your practice may be called into question and ultimately replaced with 9,9 assumptions.

Closing the Sale. Informed consent can take on the trappings of closing a sales deal. If the hard sell and the signature on the consent form give you a sense of having won something, then a red flag should go up. True informed consent comes through the patient not simply agreeing to therapy but understanding the therapy you have described and his or her own role in the treatment plan that you have developed together. There is no need to praise the patient for making "the right decision," as it is a decision you have reached as a team.

"Are There any White Flags or Other Indications That I am Moving Toward A 9,9-Oriented Medical Practice?"

Is becoming the 9,9 physician an idealistic aspiration beyond the reach of mere mortals? The answer is a resounding, "no." Although the concerted effort it takes to achieve a 9,9 orientation may seem beyond your grasp, persistence will ultimately open new doors to becoming more versatile, creative, and individualized in your approach to the art and science of medicine. Progress toward 9,9 will come in fits and starts, but you will begin to recognize signs that you are developing a 9,9 medical practice. These should reinforce your resolve and assure you that you are on the path to a more rewarding medical practice.

Increasing Patient Confidence

The 9,9 orientation gives a physician such versatility that you can immediately engage the patient and begin to build trust. Moving beyond the problem and finding a solution that fits the unique requirements of your patient build confidence that you understand the patient and are committed to meeting his or her needs.

Using the physician-patient interview to gather all the pertinent information about the medical-technical needs of the patient as well as the impact of human emotions on this situation promotes realistic expectations with regard to the medical plan. All this generates the patient's respect and appreciation for your caring and competence. The result is that patient confidence is heightened and any doubts that might lead to reluctance to cooperate are reduced.

Finding Fewer Patients Difficult

Most patients are difficult because interactions with physicians are stressful and bring out behaviors that become barriers to good care. The 9,9 physician style is most likely to produce the best outcome with these patients, because this approach stands the greatest chance of bringing a 9,9 response out in the patient. The potential for a good outcome and for the patient participating in the plan of care is enhanced by a 9,9 interaction. The white flag is recognizing that difficult patients begin to participate, build good relationships with you, and are no longer perceived as difficult.

Realizing that You Get Consistently Good Results

Several conditions come together in creating the best possible outcome. One is the consistently positive environment created when the entire team, including the patient, has thorough knowledge, clear goals, and strong convictions. Effective decision making and sound conflict solving are basic to the plan. When "who does what with whom" is made explicit, then 1/0, 1/1, and 1/all decision making are possible. Sound critique is expected, and the human resources of the team and the patient are developed to their fullest advantage. The result is that complications are reduced to a minimum, and the team is motivated to consistently strive for excellence.

Feeling Creative Energy in Place of the Dull Weight of Routine

A high level of creativity results when effective teamwork leads to synergy. The achievements of the team are greater than what the individual can accomplish alone, but more than that, the process generates a high level of energy. Open communication means that doctors, medical team members, and patients get all of their ideas out into the open, where they can be challenged or clarified. Free inquiry ensures that the real problem has the maximum likelihood of being identified. Creative decision making embodies the assessment of many different approaches for solving a problem before final action is taken. Imaginative initiative allows new ideas and changes of direction to be introduced along the way. Unconstrained conflict solving permits differences to surface, and yet, through the direct confrontation of the feelings associated with them, to avoid antagonism in resolving them. Open critique provides the means of learning how to increase effectiveness in efforts to achieve the best medical outcomes. The white flag is that the process of providing care is energized with a creativity that many thought was gone from medicine for good.

Feeling a New Sense of Satisfaction

A 9,9-oriented physician or patient gains fulfillment from contributions that make a difference in the delivery of medical care. Satisfaction is more likely to be long lasting, as it is a personal element that survives within an era of high technology. The likely result is enhanced self-esteem. In an era of public criticism and high litigation risk, increased self-esteem has a direct impact on career satisfaction, which is essential if the physician is to continue to strive for excellence.

Being a Success Beyond the Dollars and Cents of a "Busy Practice"

Evidence from research confirms that individuals within a wide variety of careers are most successful if they lead others in a 9,9 way. 9,9-oriented physicians are characterized by their peers and patients as the most reliable and capable of providing the best medical care in all situations. Consequently, the 9,9 physician achieves success from quality time with quality patients, not from the need to contract services to survive. When you, the physician, know that you have the power to make all of the difference, that incontrovertible conviction is a sign that you are well on the way to building a 9,9 practice that will endure.

Selected Bibliography

Argyris C: *Increasing Leadership Effectiveness.* New York, John Wiley and Sons, 1976.

Argyris C, Schon DA: *Theory In Practice: Increasing Professional Effectiveness.* San Francisco, Jossey-Bass, 1974.

Barr JK, Steinberg MK: A physician role typology: Colleague and client dependence in an HMO. *Soc Sci Med* 1985;20:253-261.

Bartlett EE, Grayson M, Barker R, et al.: The effects of physician communications skills on patient satisfaction, recall, and adherence. *Chronic Dis* 1984;37:755-764.

Berwick DM, Godrey AB: *Curing Health Care.* San Francisco, Jossey-Bass, 1990.

Blake RR, Mouton JS: *The Managerial Grid III.* Houston, Gulf Publishing, 1985.

Blake RR, Mouton JS, Tomaino L, et al.: *The Social Worker Grid.* Springfield, IL, Charles C. Thomas, 1979.

Blake RR, Mouton JS: *Grid Approaches to Managing Stress.* Springfield, IL, Charles C. Thomas, 1980.

Blake RR, Mouton JS, Tapper M: *Grid Approaches for Managerial Leadership in Nursing.* St. Louis, C. V. Mosby, 1981.

Blake RR, Mouton JS: A comparative analysis of situationalism and 9,9 management by principle. *Organizational Dynamics* 1982;10:20-43.

Blake RR, Mouton JS: *Solving Costly Organizational Conflicts: Achieving Intergroup Trust, Cooperation, and Teamwork.* San Francisco, Jossey-Bass, 1984.

Charles SC, Kennedy E: *Defendant: A Psychiatrist on Trial for Medical Malpractice.* New York, The Free Press, 1985.

DiMatteo MR, Linn LS, Chang BL, et al.: Affect and neutrality in physician behavior: A study of patients' values and satisfaction. *Behav Med* 1985;8:397-409.

Evans BJ, Kiellerup FD, Stanley RO, et al.: A communication skills programme for increasing patients' satisfaction with general practice consultations. *Br J Med Psychol* 1987;60:373-378.

Ewan C: Objectives for medical education: Expectations of society. *Med Educ* 1985;19:101-112.

Fiedler FE: A contingency model of leadership effectiveness. In Berkowitz L (ed): *Advances in Experimental and Social Psychology.* New York, Academic Press, 1964;1:149-190.

Fleishman EA: Leadership opinion questionnaire. Chicago, Science Research Associates, 1960.

Fleishman EA: Twenty years of consideration and structure. In Fleishman EA, Hunt JG (eds): *Current Developments in the Study of Leadership.* Carbondale, IL, Southern Illinois University Press, 1973;1-40.

Gaucher EJ, Coffey RJ: *Total Quality in Healthcare.* San Francisco, Jossey-Bass, 1993.

Greenfield S, Kaplan S, Ware JW Jr: Expanding patient involvement in care. Effects on patient outcomes. *Ann Intern Med* 1985;102:520-528.

Hersey PG, Blanchard KH: *Management of Organizational Behavior: Utilizing Human Resources,* 4th ed. Englewood Cliffs, NJ, Prentice-Hall, 1982.

Horn S, Hopkins DSP: *Clinical Practice Improvement: A New Technology for Developing Cost-Effective Quality Health Care, Volume 1.* Faulkner & Gray, Inc. New York, 1994.

House RJ: A path-goal theory of leadership effectiveness. *Admin Sci Q* 1971;16:321-338.

Jackson D: United Airlines' Cockpit Resource Management training. In *Proceedings of the Second Symposium on Aviation Psychology.* Columbus, OH, Ohio State University, April 25-28, 1983.

Kantor RM: *The Change Masters.* New York, Simon and Schuster, 1983.

Kipnis D, Schmidt SM, Swaffin-Smith C., et al.: Patterns of managerial influence: Shotgun managers, tacticians, and bystanders. *Organizational Dynamics* 1984; (Winter):

Korzybski A: *Science and Sanity, An Introduction to Non-Aristotelian Systems and General Semantics,* 4th ed. Lakeville, CT, International Non-Aristotelian Library Publishing, 1958.

Korzybski A, Kendig M: Foreword. In *A Theory of Meaning Analyzed.* Lakeville, CT, International Non-Aristotelian Library Publishing, General Semantics Monograph III, 1942.

Lefton RE, Buzzotta VR, Sherberg M: *Improving Productivity Through People Skills.* Cambridge, MA, Ballinger Publishing Company, 1980.

Ley P: Doctor-patient communication: Some quantitative estimates of the role of cognitive factors in non-compliance. *Hypertension* 1985;3(Suppl):S51-S55.

Like R, Zyzanski SJ: Patient satisfaction with the clinical encounter: Social psychological determinants. *Soc Sci Med* 1987;24:351-357.

Likert RG: *The Human Organization: Its Management and Value.* New York, McGraw-Hill, 1967.

Likert RG, Likert JG: *New Ways of Managing Conflict.* New York, McGraw-Hill, 1976.

Linn LS, DiMatteo MR, Chang BL, et al.: Consumer values and subsequent satisfaction ratings of physician behavior. *Med Care* 1984;22:804-812.

Maccoby M: *The Gamesman.* New York, Simon and Schuster, 1976. Maccoby M: *The Leader.* New York, Simon and Schuster, 1981.

McGregor D: *The Human Side of Enterprise.* New York, McGraw-Hill, 1960.

Mouton JS, Blake RR: *Synergogy: A New Strategy for Education, Training, and Development.* San Francisco, Jossey-Bass, 1984.

Odiorne G: *The Change Resisters.* Englewood Cliffs, NJ, Prentice-Hall, 1981.

Pascale RT, Athos A: *The Art of Japanese Management*. New York, Simon and Schuster, 1981.

Peters TJ, Waterman RH Jr: *In Search of Excellence*. New York, Harper and Row, 1982.

Schutz W: *The Schutz Measures: An Integrated System for Assessing Elements of Awareness*. San Diego, University Associates, 1984.

Service ER: *Origins of the State and Civilization*. New York, W. W. Norton, 1975.

Shapiro MC, Najman JM, Chang A, et al.: Information control and the exercise of power in the obstetrical encounter. *Soc Sci Med* 1983;17:139-146.

Speedling EJ, Rose DN: Building an effective doctor-patient relationship: From patient satisfaction to patient participation. *Soc Sci Med* 1985;21:115-120.

Stewart MA: What is a successful doctor-patient interview? A study of interactions and outcomes. *Soc Sci Med* 1984;19:167-175.

Vroom VH, Yetton PW: *Leadership and Decision-Making*. Pittsburgh, University of Pittsburgh Press, 1973.

Waitzkin H: Doctor-patient communication. Clinical implications of social scientific research. *JAMA* 1984;252:2441-2446.

Weisman CS, Teitelbaum MA: Physician gender and the physician-patient relationship: Recent evidence and relevant questions. *Soc Sci Med* 1985;20:1119-1127.

Zweig S, Kruse J, LeFevre M: Patient satisfaction with obstetric care. *J Family Prac* 1986;23:131-136.

Index